Handbook of
Minimally Invasive and Percutaneous Spine Surgery

Handbook of
Minimally Invasive and Percutaneous Spine Surgery

Edited by

Michael Y. Wang, MD, FACS
Associate Professor, Departments of
Neurological Surgery and Rehabilitation Medicine,
University of Miami Miller School of Medicine,
Miami, Florida

D. Greg Anderson, MD
Associate Professor, Department of Orthopaedic Surgery,
Thomas Jefferson University, Philadelphia, Pennsylvania

Steven C. Ludwig, MD
Associate Professor and Chief of Spine Surgery;
Fellowship Director, Department of Orthopaedics,
University of Maryland School of Medicine,
Baltimore, Maryland

Praveen V. Mummaneni, MD
Associate Professor, Department of Neurosurgery; Co-Director,
University of California–San Francisco Spine Center,
San Francisco, California

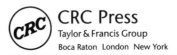

CRC Press
Taylor & Francis Group
Boca Raton London New York

CRC Press is an imprint of the
Taylor & Francis Group, an **informa** business

CRC Press
Taylor & Francis Group
6000 Broken Sound Parkway NW, Suite 300
Boca Raton, FL 33487-2742

© 2011 by Taylor & Francis Group, LLC
CRC Press is an imprint of Taylor & Francis Group, an Informa business

Visit the Taylor & Francis Web site at
http://www.taylorandfrancis.com

and the CRC Press Web site at
http://www.crcpress.com

For Amy, Patrick, Evan, and Sarah
M.Y.W.

To my wife, Sandra, for supporting my academic work
D.G.A.

To my wife, Cindy, and children, Ethan and Katie,
for their never-ending love and support
S.C.L.

For my wife, Valli, and my children,
for their love and support

Also for my residents and fellows,
whose hard work I admire on a daily basis
P.V.M.

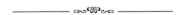

Contributors

D. Greg Anderson, MD
Associate Professor, Department of Orthopaedic Surgery,
Thomas Jefferson University, Philadelphia, Pennsylvania

Kelley E. Banagan, MD
Orthopaedic Spine Fellow, Department of Orthopaedic Surgery,
Rush University Medical Center, Chicago, Illinois

Sanjay S. Dhall, MD
Assistant Professor, Department of Neurosurgery, Emory
University School of Medicine; Chief of Neurosurgery,
Department of Neurosurgery, Grady Memorial Hospital,
Atlanta, Georgia

Florian F. Dibra, BS
Medical Student Year 3, Jefferson Medical College,
Philadelphia, Pennsylvania

Robert W. Irwin, MD
Associate Professor, Department of Rehabilitation Medicine,
University of Miami Miller School of Medicine, Miami, Florida

Steven C. Ludwig, MD
Associate Professor and Chief of Spine Surgery; Fellowship
Director, Department of Orthopaedics, University of Maryland
School of Medicine, Baltimore, Maryland

Praveen V. Mummaneni, MD
Associate Professor, Department of Neurosurgery;
Co-Director, University of California–San Francisco Spine Center,
San Francisco, California

Philip R. Neubauer, RPh, MD
Assistant Professor, Department of Orthopedics,
Johns Hopkins University Hospital, Baltimore, Maryland

Andrew C. Roeser, MD
Department of Neurosurgery, The Methodist Hospital,
Houston, Texas

Amirali Sayadipour, MD
Department of Orthopaedic Surgery, Rothman Institute at
Thomas Jefferson University, Philadelphia, Pennsylvania

Jason S. Taub, MD
Senior Resident, Department of Neurosurgery,
Emory University School of Medicine, Atlanta, Georgia

Michael Y. Wang, MD, FACS
Associate Professor, Departments of Neurological Surgery
and Rehabilitation Medicine, University of Miami Miller
School of Medicine, Miami, Florida

Foreword

Doctors Wang, Anderson, Ludwig, and Mummaneni have created a unique educational manual that is focused, comprehensive, and well organized. This is perhaps at least partly because every chapter is authored by one of the editors, each of whom is well known and highly respected in the field of minimally invasive spine surgery. The text specifically considers only two topics: minimally invasive lumbar fusion and percutaneous pedicle screw fixation. Because of this, the text manages to be thorough without being exhausting, and focused without being irrelevant.

The unique nature of this text is immediately obvious on reviewing the list of chapters. It begins with the true foundation of minimally invasive surgery: imaging. Safe and effective surgery performed through minimal exposures demands a thorough mind's-eye understanding of anatomy without its visualization. Moreover, it requires a keen ability to mentally translate two-dimensional imaging into three-dimensional anatomy. The importance of these two traits is emphasized in this text by its devotion of four chapters to these topics. Chapter 2 introduces the relationship between imaging and anatomy, and details the problems that can arise if attention is not paid to magnification, distortion, and parallax. The two most common techniques of cannulation are covered in a logical, step-by-step fashion, just as it would be taught to residents in the operating room. Chapter 1, however, is unique. Even before the concepts and techniques of fluoroscopically guided pedicle screw insertion are covered, the risks of radiation exposure are discussed, along with techniques to minimize exposure. Finally, minimally invasive options for pedicle screw placement are completed with the description of a mini-open technique in Chapter 5. Not only can mini-open techniques reduce exposure to radiation, but they also provide a somewhat easier, intermediate step for surgeons transitioning between traditional open surgery and fully minimally invasive surgery.

During the past 5 years, minimally invasive spine surgery techniques have seen significant evolution. The second half of this book discusses these advances while maintaining its focus on fusion and pedicle screw insertion. As our experience, skill level, and instrumentation systems have evolved, minimally invasive surgery has taken on increasingly more complex problems, such as trauma, multilevel degenerative disease, and complex spinal deformity. In this context, the most recent technique for interbody fusion (direct lateral), is described in detail in Chapter 6, after which its necessary counterpart, multilevel minimally invasive rod passage, is discussed in Chapter 7. Because these cases truly can be challenging, important tips for successfully cannulating the pedicles is discussed in Chapter 10, followed by a concluding chapter aptly titled "Pushing the Limits." Finally, this handbook does not ignore the endpoint of all these techniques: achieving successful fusion. Techniques to enhance the success of this outcome are discussed in Chapter 9, whereas potential complications and methods to help avoid them are discussed in Chapter 8.

Readers will find the "Surgical Pearls and Pitfalls" in each chapter to be excellent summaries of the salient points discussed in that chapter, and they are highlighted to make them easy to find for quick reference and review. Unique to this text, however, is the highlighted table detailing "Bailouts/Alternative Strategies" for completing the task when classic techniques fail. This is a particularly useful feature for any surgeon. Furthermore, each chapter is well illustrated, with images that clearly demonstrate the points being made.

I believe any reader will find this text well worth the investment. For residents and novices of minimally invasive surgery, it provides the basics to safely get started in minimally invasive fusion and pedicle screw insertion. For surgeons with more experience, the pearls, pitfalls, and bailouts will augment their knowledge and confidence. All of this is achieved, moreover, in a concise and readable format.

Richard G. Fessler, MD, PhD
Professor, Feinberg School of Medicine,
Northwestern University, Chicago, Illinois

Foreword

Minimally invasive spine surgery is at a crossroads. Every spine surgeon wants to improve patient outcomes and reduce complications and postoperative pain. Many surgeons have attempted minimally invasive approaches but have soon become discouraged because of the technical difficulty, prolonged surgical times, excessive complications during the initial learning phase, or concerns about radiation exposure. The superior clinical results, equivalent operative times, and reduced complications of the most experienced minimally invasive spine surgeons have not been consistently replicated by those who are less experienced. This discrepancy becomes greater as more complicated surgical procedures such as deformity correction and tumor resection are attempted. Without a way to jump-start the learning process, minimally invasive approaches will likely continue to be restricted to a few extremely experienced surgeons and those trainees who spend long periods of mentorship during residency or fellowship.

The *Handbook of Minimally Invasive and Percutaneous Spine Surgery* presents the distilled technical knowledge and experience of a select group of world-recognized minimally invasive spine surgeons. This handbook provides important practical details needed to safely and effectively perform minimally invasive procedures. There is a particular focus on guiding surgeons with experience in performing open spine surgery to convert to less invasive approaches. Many useful tips include the subtleties of obtaining ideal radiographic images, optimizing the starting point for the surgical procedure, minimizing patient and surgeon radiation exposure, overcoming the difficulty of passing the rod percutaneously through the screw extenders, and methods of achieving a successful fusion. As a less experienced minimally invasive surgeon, I was immediately provided with numerous ways to improve my surgical technique and overcome areas of frustration. This handbook also provides helpful information on reducing side effects and complications unique to minimally invasive approaches such as management of postoperative muscle spasms.

This handbook fills a large void that has existed in the education of both trainees and experienced spine surgeons. Until now, the primary way for orthopedic or neurosurgery residents and fellows to learn the details of minimally invasive techniques was through a mentorship process with an experienced minimally invasive spine surgeon in the operating room. Although nothing can fully substitute for hands-on training, this handbook does provide an extremely valuable framework to permit a much more safe and rapid learning experience.

This outstanding distillation of years of practical experience into an easily readable and immediately useful manual appeals to spine surgeons at all levels. Residents and fellows are presented with state-of-the-art techniques in a straightforward style. For established practitioners making the transition from open to minimally invasive spine surgery, this handbook gives the technical details to markedly reduce the learning curve inherent in the transition from open to minimally invasive approaches. Even those with considerable minimally invasive spine surgery experience will find this handbook useful, because the techniques of this evolving field are not standardized, and learning the tricks and approaches of other experts can be invaluable.

Christopher I. Shaffrey, MD, FACS
Harrison Distinguished Professor,
Department of Neurological and Orthopaedic Surgery,
University of Virginia, Charlottesville, Virginia

Preface

In the past decade we have witnessed a renaissance in spine surgery. Great enthusiasm has been expressed by both physicians and patients for more minimally invasive techniques for treating spinal instability with fewer sequelae. This enthusiasm has led to the development of diverse technologies for introducing percutaneous implants to treat the thoracolumbar spine.

As surgical specialists who treat disorders of the spinal column, we have become convinced of the potential advantages of minimally invasive approaches in select patients. Each of us has set out to identify, refine, and perfect surgical techniques for treating difficult spine cases. Our experiences with learning these new techniques have come with great challenges and trials, but have led to a better way to perform percutaneous spinal stabilization.

The four editors of this book began discussing some of these new strategies at national meetings, and our shared ideas and concepts were significantly improved by these interactions. Many other surgeons also participated in these discussions, and to them we owe a debt of gratitude for helping us improve our techniques. What became abundantly clear throughout this process was that there was no one superior technique, and that the surgical methods were undergoing a rapid evolution. It was also clear that many surgeons (both those in training and those with decades of experience) were, in effect, each reinventing the wheel. The learning curve was steep as we attempted to perform these surgeries more efficiently and with greater efficacy. In the process, surgeons performing minimally invasive procedures were receiving more radiation exposure and subjecting themselves to increased physical demands. Furthermore, as each of us trained residents and fellows in our respective institutions, we saw the reinvention process played out over and over again.

The end result of these factors is this *Handbook of Minimally Invasive and Percutaneous Spine Surgery.* We wanted to create an easy-to-access source of written information that would provide surgeons with an overview of all the major minimally invasive and mini-open procedures, including lateral lumbar interbody fusion, TLIF, and percutaneous screws, as well as shortcuts and bailouts for both common and esoteric problems that might be encountered. Although we are sure that some of the suggestions offered here are obvious or controversial, we hope that you, the reader, will be able to glean some elements that will improve your surgical techniques. No doubt, some elements of this handbook will be obsolete in time, but as together we move through this evolutionary period in spinal surgery, we hope that this book will serve as a starting or turning point for you.

We see the spine surgery community as a collective. Orthopedic and neurologic surgeons alike have a vested interest in improving outcomes for our patients. If you, the reader, are able to offer an advanced tip or trick to us, or to any other spine surgeon (maybe as a result of something you read in this handbook), then this endeavor will be considered a great success!

Michael Y. Wang
D. Greg Anderson
Steven C. Ludwig
Praveen V. Mummaneni

Contents

Handbook of
Minimally Invasive and Percutaneous Spine Surgery

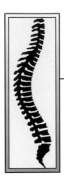

1

Intraoperative Imaging: Radiation Safety, Techniques, and Technology

Florian F. Dibra, D. Greg Anderson,
Amirali Sayadipour

Minimally invasive or minimal access spinal surgery is, as the name suggests, performed with minimal direct exposure of the spinal anatomy. Because of the complex topography of the spine and its close proximity to neurologic and vital structures, a high degree of positional awareness is necessary throughout all aspects of the surgical procedure. Therefore, a minimally invasive spine surgeon must rely on intraoperative imaging to provide information on the location of anatomic landmarks at key points during the procedure.

Intraoperative imaging options include radiographic techniques such as plain radiographs, two-dimensional fluoroscopy using a portable C-arm or O-arm, computed tomography using a specialized C-arm or O-arm, image guidance technologies, or robotic technologies. Many of these technologies are relatively recent or still in a developmental stage.

RADIATION SAFETY

Imaging modalities that depend on the use of x-rays, such as plain radiography and fluoroscopy, produce ionizing radiation that has a potential negative impact on human health. Various units have been developed to measure the amount of ionizing radiation delivered from these medical imaging and therapy sources.[1] When assessing the risk of ionizing radiation, the preferred unit is the sievert (Sv). A sievert is defined as a 1 joule per kilogram of body tissue, averaged over the whole body. The sievert is similar to the gray, except that the latter is not weighted to specific body tissues. In occupational settings, radiation is measured in millisieverts (mSv), or 1/1000 Sv. The average effective dose of ionizing radiation to each person in the United States during 2006 was 6.2 mSv.[2] Much of this exposure (37%) was from radon and thoron gases, which can accumulate in basements. Medical sources accounted for 48% of the annual exposure.

Medical professionals are considered radiation workers by the United States Occupational Safety and Health Administration (OSHA). The National Council on Radiation Protection (NCRP) and the International Commission on Radiologic Protection (ICRP) issue annual reports advising on maximum annual radiation doses for radiation workers. The annual exposure limit given by both organizations is 50 mSv per year.[3,4] The NCRP and ICRP recommendations are included in Box 1-1.

It is important to know that radiation exposure does not have a threshold effect, which means that there is no dose of radiation below which the risk of excess tumor formation is zero. In addition, the effects of radiation exposure are cumulative over the course of a lifetime. Also, human studies have demonstrated a roughly linear relationship between radiation exposure and cancer risk. Previous studies have shown that a single radiation exposure above 100 mSv increases the risk of some cancers in humans.[5] One study

Box 1-1
Annual Radiation Exposure Limits
Set by the NCRP and ICRP

Occupational Exposures

Annual effective dose limit:	50 mSv per year
Cumulative effective dose limit:	10 mSv × age (years)

Equivalent Dose Limits for Specific Tissues

Lens of eye:	150 mSv
Skin, hands, feet:	500 mSv
Thyroid:	20 mSv

Compiled from Balter S. An overview of radiation safety regulatory recommendations and requirements. Catheter Cardiovasc Interv 47:469-474, 1999; and Jones DP, Robertson PA, Lunt B, et al. Radiation exposure during fluoroscopically assisted pedicle screw insertion in the lumbar spine. Spine 25:1538-1541, 2000.

documented an increased rate of DNA translocations and certain cancers in airline pilots, who are exposed to radiation from flying at high altitudes.[6] The risk of cancer was found to increase with more years of flight, demonstrating the cumulative effect of this occupational radiation.

Orthopaedic surgeons have been shown to have a five-fold increased chance of tumor development compared with other hospital workers, presumably caused by the prolonged occupational exposure to ionizing radiation.[7] Using the C-arm during lumbar pedicle screw placement has been shown to produce 10 to 12 times the radiation exposure of nonspinal musculoskeletal procedures involving fluoroscopy.[8] Patient exposure is also important to consider. One study demonstrated that a lumbar instrumented fusion with fluoroscopic assistance exposes patients to an average entry dose of 43 mSv (range: 18 to 107 mSv), which is 6.9 times the av-

Table 1-1
Relative Radiation Exposure of Common
Diagnostic Imaging Modalities

Modality	Radiation Exposure to Patient (mSv)
Lumbar AP and lateral radiograph	1.8
Fluoroscopic insertion of percutaneous pedicle screw (0.33 minute of exposure)	0.5
Fluoroscopic insertion of single level percutaneous pedicle screw construct (1.4 minutes of exposure)	2.3
Spiral CT scan of chest or abdomen	10-20
Cardiac ablation procedure	10-300

erage annual effective dose.[9] The relative radiation exposure of various imaging modalities is shown in Table 1-1.

In addition to the risk of cancer, radiation exposure can cause cataract formation in the posterior capsular region of the eye. Cataracts have been shown to occur 4.6 times more frequently in radiation workers than in nonradiation workers.[10,11] In a prospective study of 27 patients who underwent kyphoplasty, radiation exposure to the eye was 0.271 ± 0.200 mSv per vertebra when eye shields were not used.[12] Because the exact dose of radiation necessary to induce cataract formation is not known, it is important for the surgical team to use proper eye protection during every case in which fluoroscopy is employed. Eye protection is obtained in the form of leaded glasses with an equivalent of 0.75 mm of lead protection, and they are available from a variety of commercial sources.

The primary source of radiation exposure in the operating room is the C-arm fluoroscopy unit. When using the C-arm, most of the radiation that reaches the surgeon and the medical team has been deflected by tissues and other solid objects in the path of the beam. Fortunately, some relatively simple measures can significantly limit the exposure of the medical team to ionizing radiation. First, personal protective equipment is essential for the surgical team during every case in which fluoroscopy is used. Adequate protective equipment includes a leaded apron (0.5 mm of lead equivalent), leaded glasses (0.75 mm of lead equivalent), and a thyroid shield (0.5 mm of lead equivalent). Second, the use of fluoroscopy should be kept to a minimum during the procedure. Radiation scatter, and therefore exposure, is significantly less when standing on the side of the imager rather than on the side of the radiation source. Therefore, when possible, the surgeon should stand away from the source when using cross-table imaging. When obtaining anteroposterior images, placing the radiation source inferior to the patient with the image intensifier surface as close as possible to the patient's back produces the least radiation exposure to the surgical team.[9] Other methods to limit radiation exposure include using tight collimation of the fluoroscopic beam and avoiding the magnification mode. The surgeon should always keep his or her hands away from the beam and stand back from the table when possible during fluoroscopic imaging. The surgeon also should use spot images rather than continuous fluoroscopy whenever possible. Finally, certain techniques for pedicle screw insertion can significantly limit the fluoroscopic beam time during pedicle screw insertion (see Chapter 5).

TECHNIQUES AND TECHNOLOGIES

The primary imaging modality used in the operating room during minimally invasive spinal surgery is the C-arm image intensifier fluoroscope. The C-arm image intensifier uses a cesium iodide phosphor deposited directly on a photocathode in the intensifier tube to brighten the raw fluoroscopic image by a factor of 10.[9] An advantage of the C-arm is the fact that this portable unit is readily available in most hospital operating rooms and is able to provide quick, real-time images throughout the surgical procedure. Disadvantages of the C-arm include the requirement of a skilled technician to operate the equipment during surgery, the exposure to ionizing radiation, and the bulkiness of the equipment, which can be difficult to work around. Also, some surgeons find that wearing a leaded apron is quite uncomfortable during surgery.

Other imaging modalities include units that provide computed tomography-like images, including the Iso-C C-arm from Siemens (Erlangen, Germany) and the O-arm from Medtronic Sofamor Danek USA (Memphis, TN) (Fig. 1-1). These units can provide two-dimensional fluoroscopic images like a conventional C-arm, or can provide cross-sectional images in various planes by taking multiple fluoroscopic shots in a circle around the patient. This allows the surgeon to evaluate axial images, which are especially advantageous in defining the position of a pedicle screw relative to the spinal canal. Also, these units can be fitted with image guidance equipment, allowing the surgeon to perform image-guided surgery. Disadvantages of this type of equipment include the ionizing radiation along with the relative bulk and higher cost of the equipment.

Image-guided surgery is performed by fitting the patient's spine and surgical instruments with tracking devices that allow a computer system to track the relative position in three-dimensional

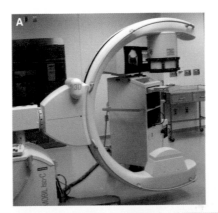

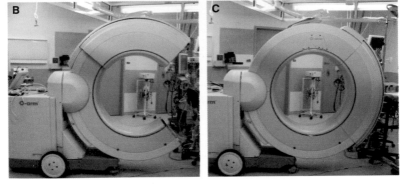

FIG. 1-1   A, An isocentric C-arm can obtain standard two-dimensional fluoroscopic images and tomographic images reformatted in various planes. B and C, The O-arm in the open and closed positions. The O-arm can be used for standard two-dimensional fluoroscopic images and can take high-quality tomographic images reformatted in various planes.

space of the instruments and the spine, and provide a visual illustration of the relationship by showing the virtual position of the instruments on preacquired spinal images. The types of images most commonly used for image-guided surgery include fluoroscopic images and CT images. The images may be acquired before surgery and loaded into the image guidance computer, or may be obtained at the beginning of the procedure using a C-arm or related equipment such as an O-arm. Advantages of image guidance systems are the relative reduction in ionizing radiation and the ability to evaluate the position of instruments relative to spinal images throughout the procedure. Disadvantages of image guidance include the bulk, high cost, and complexity of these systems. In addition, the tracking devices can be bumped during surgery, with a resulting loss of locational accuracy.

CONCLUSION

Understanding radiation exposure and the diagnostic imaging modalities currently available for use during surgery enhances the safety of minimally invasive spine surgeons and improves surgical outcomes.

SURGICAL PEARLS AND PITFALLS

- Use personal protective equipment, including a leaded apron (0.5 mm of lead equivalent), leaded glasses (0.75 mm of lead equivalent), and a thyroid shield (0.5 mm of lead equivalent).

- Fluoroscopy use should be kept to a minimum during the procedure.

- When possible, the surgeon should stand away from the radiation source when using cross-table imaging.

- When obtaining anteroposterior images, placing the radiation source inferior to the patient and the image intensifier surface as close as possible to the patient's back produces the least radiation.

- Use tight collimation of the fluoroscopic beam and avoid the magnification mode.

- Always keep hands away from the beam and stand back from the table when possible during fluoroscopic imaging.

- Use spot images rather than continuous fluoroscopy whenever possible.

- Use techniques for pedicle screw insertion that limit the fluoroscopic beam time.

- New technologies, such as image guidance systems, can limit the surgical team's exposure to ionizing radiation.

References

1. Grover SB, Kumar J. A review of the current concepts of radiation measurement and its biological effects. Indian J Radiol Imaging 12: 21-32, 2002. Available at *www.ijri.org/text.asp?2002/12/1/21/28413*.
2. The National Council on Radiation Protection and Measurements. Ionizing Radiation Exposure of the Population of the United States, 2009. Available at *www.ncrppublications.org/Reports/160*.
3. Giordano BD, Baumhauer JF, Morgan TL, et al. Cervical spine imaging using standard C-arm fluoroscopy. Spine 33:1970-1976, 2008.
4. Balter S. An overview of radiation safety regulatory recommendations and requirements. Catheter Cardiovasc Interv 47:469-474, 1999.
5. Brenner DJ, Doll R, Goodhead DT, et al. Cancer risks attributable to low doses of ionizing radiation: assessing what we really know. Proc Natl Acad Sci USA 100:13761-13766, 2003.
6. Yong LC, Sigurdson AJ, Ward EM, et al. Increased frequency of chromosome translocations in airline pilots with long-term flying experience. Occup Environ Med 66:56-62, 2009.
7. Mastrangelo G, Fedeli U, Fadda E. Increased cancer risk among surgeons in an orthopaedic hospital. Occup Med 55:498-500, 2005.
8. Kim CW, Lee YP, Taylor W, et al. Use of navigation-assisted fluoroscopy to decrease radiation exposure during minimally invasive spine surgery. Spine J 8:584-590, 2008.
9. Jones DP, Robertson PA, Lunt B, et al. Radiation exposure during fluoroscopically assisted pedicle screw insertion in the lumbar spine. Spine 25:1538-1541, 2000.
10. Milacic S. Risk of occupational radiation-induced cataract in medical workers. Med Lav 100:178-186, 2009.
11. Ainsbury EA, Bouffler SD, Dörr W, et al. Radiation cataractogenesis: a review of recent studies. Radiat Res 172:1-9, 2009.
12. Mroz TE, Yamashita T, Davros WJ, et al. Radiation exposure to the surgeon and the patient during kyphoplasty. J Spinal Disord Tech 21:96-100, 2008.

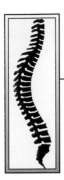

2

Anatomic Relationships With Two-Dimensional Imaging

Philip R. Neubauer, Florian F. Dibra,
D. Greg Anderson

When a surgeon is performing percutaneous spinal fixation, his or her ability to use and interpret fluoroscopic images is essential to the success of the procedure.

IMAGE MAGNIFICATION, DISTORTION, AND PARALLAX

Fluoroscopic images are subject to various types of distortion that must be understood to successfully use the C-arm mobile image intensifier. The most common types of image inaccuracies are magnification, distortion, and parallax. These image misrepresentations occur because x-rays emanate from a point source and are focused into a relative beam by the x-ray tube. The x-ray beams are partially absorbed by the imaged tissue, and the nonabsorbed x-rays reach a detector surface (Fig. 2-1, *A*). However, the paths of individual x-rays are not parallel but rather slightly divergent as they leave the x-ray tube and travel toward the image detector surface (the image intensifier when using a C-arm) (Fig. 2-1, *B*). X-rays traveling at the edges of the x-ray tube have a larger divergence angle than x-rays in the central region of the tube. These fundamental aspects of x-ray imaging produce certain image inaccuracies that must be anticipated and understood.

Magnification occurs because the x-rays travel on a divergent path, passing through the imaged tissue before reaching the de-

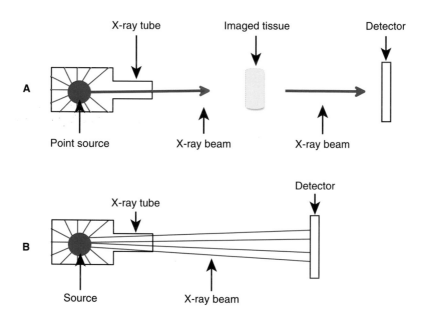

FIG. 2-1 **A,** Diagnostic imaging setup for a radiographic image. **B,** X-ray beam divergence.

tector surface. This produces an image that is larger than the actual tissue of interest (Fig. 2-2, *A*). Image magnification is more significant when the imaged tissue is closer to the x-ray source and farther from the image detector surface (Fig. 2-2, *B*). Magnification may be desirable in some instances to enhance anatomic detail during a percutaneous procedure. If magnification is desired, the C-arm should be adjusted to move the vertebra closer to the x-ray source. In other situations, it is more desirable to see several vertebral segments within a single image. In this case, the surgeon should adjust the C-arm so that the spine is closer to the image detector surface to increase the field of view.

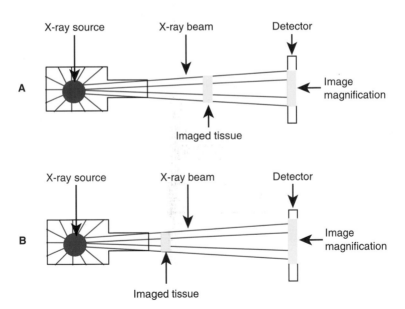

FIG. 2-2 *A*, Image magnification caused by beam divergence. *B*, Objects placed closer to the x-ray source are more magnified than objects placed farther from the source, which allows zooming in for finer detail.

Distortion occurs when the x-ray beam is not perpendicular to the vertebra of interest (Fig. 2-3, *A*). When using a C-arm, the image beam is always perpendicular to the detector surface. Distortion occurs when the C-arm beam is not aligned orthogonally to the imaged vertebra. Misalignment of the C-arm results in a skewed image that can easily be misinterpreted by the surgeon, leading to

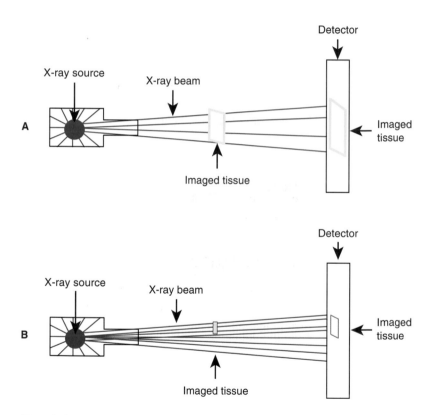

FIG. 2-3   **A**, Image distortion is caused by misalignment of the imaged tissue (vertebra) within the x-ray beam. **B**, Parallax occurs if the imaged tissue is not centered.

implant malposition. Image distortion must be recognized and corrected before using the fluoroscopic images for surgical guidance. On a lateral view of the vertebral column, distortion is seen if the pedicles are not superimposed and/or the vertebral endplates are not aligned (Fig. 2-3, *B*). On an AP image of the spine, distortion is recognized as misalignment of the endplates and/or the spinous process not being equidistant between the pedicles. In either case, the C-arm should be adjusted until an optimal image, without distortion, is achieved (Fig. 2-4).

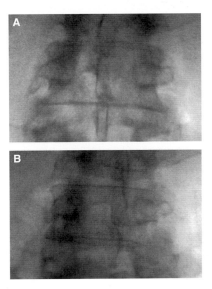

FIG. 2-4 Misaligned AP images. **A,** The x-ray beam was not parallel to the superior endplate, and two endplate shadows can be seen. **B,** Malrotated image—the spinous process is not centered.

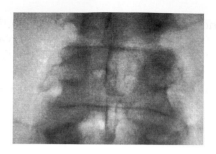

FIG. 2-5   Properly aligned AP image with the beam parallel to superior endplate. The pedicle is just inferior to the endplate, and the spinous process is centered.

Parallax is a phenomenon of viewing an object from two different vantage points and thus seeing a different relationship between objects in the foreground and the background of the image. Parallax is always produced at the edges of a C-arm image by the diverging x-ray beams, because they are not parallel to structures located at the image's edges—the divergence angle is always greatest at the edges of an image (Fig. 2-5). The effects of parallax are more significant in C-arms with a larger detector surface (such as a 12-inch detector surface rather than an 8-inch one). To avoid misinterpretation of C-arm images, the region of interest should always be positioned in the center of the image, rather than at the periphery.

USEFUL C-ARM IMAGES FOR MINIMALLY INVASIVE SURGERY

Perhaps the most useful view in minimally invasive spine surgery is a true AP image of the vertebra of interest. In a properly aligned true AP image, the center of the x-ray beam is aligned parallel to the superior endplate of the vertebra (Fig. 2-6). This produces a single (superimposed) superior endplate shadow. The pedicle shadows should be just caudal to the superior endplate shadow. The spinous process shadow should appear equidistant between the pedicle shadows. The transverse processes should be just lateral to the pedicle shadows and aligned parallel to the superior endplate shadow. A true AP image is particularly useful during cannulation of the pedicles (Fig. 2-7).

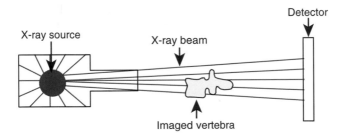

FIG. 2-6   In a true AP image, the central beam of the x-ray is parallel to the superior endplate of the imaged vertebra.

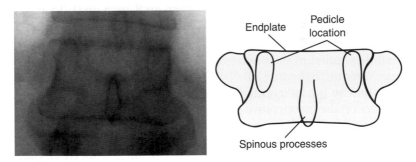

FIG. 2-7   True AP view of a vertebra. The endplate appears as a single line, the pedicles are just inferior to the endplate, and the spinous process is centered between the pedicles.

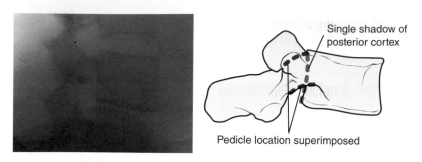

FIG. 2-8   True lateral view. The endplate shadows are superimposed and the pedicles are superimposed. The posterior cortex is also superimposed, which ensures that the image is not rotated.

A lateral image also requires proper alignment. To obtain a true lateral C-arm image, the x-ray beam is aligned parallel to the superior endplate of the vertebra, producing a single (superimposed) shadow. The pedicles' shadows (right and left) are also superimposed. In addition, the posterior cortex shows only a single (superimposed) shadow, indicating that there is no vertebral rotation (Fig. 2-8).

Another useful view for pedicle cannulation is the en face view of the pedicle (see Chapter 4). To obtain this view, the x-ray beam is aligned directly in line with the pedicle axis. The surgeon begins with a true AP image. Then the C-arm is rotated until the x-ray beam is parallel to the pedicle of interest (generally 10 to 30 degrees oblique to the true AP view) (Fig. 2-9). The exact amount of rotation can be determined by measuring the angulation of the pedicles on the preoperative imaging study. Alternatively, the C-arm is generally well-aligned with the pedicle axis when the medial margin of the superior articular process aligns with the medial wall of the pedicle on the image.

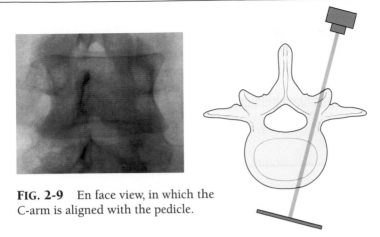

FIG. 2-9   En face view, in which the C-arm is aligned with the pedicle.

LIMITATIONS OF TWO-DIMENSIONAL IMAGES

Properly aligned AP and lateral images are essential for a surgeon to safely perform most percutaneous procedures on the vertebral column. However, the axial image (obtained with a CT scan or MRI) is not available with two-dimensional imaging. Thus it may not be possible to detect small breaches of the medial wall of the pedicle when placing pedicle screw implants very close to this structure. For this reason, it is best to keep the implants a few millimeters away from the medial wall of the pedicle to ensure that no minor pedicle breach may be missed with two-dimensional imaging. For small pedicles or for situations in which it is desirable to be very close to the medial wall of the pedicle, the en face view offers a more accurate way to visualize the implant relative to the medial border of the pedicle.

CONCLUSION

Pedicles can be safely cannulated using two-dimensional imaging. It is crucial to use properly aligned images when performing percutaneous instrumentation. By understanding the characteristics of radiographic images and by giving proper attention to details, a surgeon can master the use of fluoroscopy during minimally invasive procedures to ensure accurate visualization of complex spinal anatomy.

SURGICAL PEARLS AND PITFALLS

- Always use properly aligned images when performing percutaneous instrumentation.

- A true AP image is the most useful view for pedicle cannulation in most situations.

- The en face view can be helpful if the pedicle anatomy is not well visualized on the true AP view.

- Avoid accepting poor-quality fluoroscopic images when performing percutaneous surgery.

- Keep in mind how parallax, distortion, and magnification can lead to poor-quality images.

BAILOUTS/ALTERNATIVE STRATEGIES

- Biplanar fluoroscopy may be useful in certain situations.

- Intraoperative O-arm imaging can be helpful to confirm the location of implants relative to the spinal canal.

- Open exposure and identification of anatomic landmarks can always be considered if adequate images cannot be obtained using fluoroscopy.

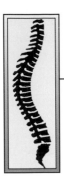

3

Pedicle Cannulation With True Anteroposterior Fluoroscopic Imaging

Philip R. Neubauer, Florian F. Dibra,
D. Greg Anderson

Pedicle screw fixation is the most common and biomechanically sound form of internal fixation used for thoracolumbar spinal pathology. Unfortunately, traditional techniques for placing pedicle screw instrumentation are invasive and involve substantial muscle stripping for exposure. Recent advances in percutaneous pedicle screw technology allow the placement of these constructs in the thoracolumbar region with less muscle trauma.

When placing percutaneous pedicle screws, the most commonly used intraoperative imaging modality is the C-arm image intensifier. The C-arm provides two-dimensional images of the bony anatomy by superimposing the shadows of all tissues traversed by the fluoroscopic beam. With experience, surgeons can locate the pedicle using a true AP view of the vertebra.

Pedicle cannulation using a true AP view has several advantages over other pedicle cannulation strategies:

- This technique is set up quickly and performed in a time-efficient manner.
- It avoids the potential loss of sterility and asepsis associated with repeatedly alternating between AP and lateral views during pedicle cannulation.
- The true AP technique allows two surgeons to work simultaneously on both sides of the spine, reducing both procedure time and radiation exposure.
- True AP images of the pedicle help obtain a high degree of accuracy in pedicle cannulation, assuming the surgeon correctly aligns the C-arm to produce the proper images and carefully performs the subsequent steps.
- This technique minimizes total radiation exposure to the patient and to the health care providers.

INDICATIONS AND CONTRAINDICATIONS

The AP pedicle cannulation technique is indicated for pedicle cannulation during the placement of percutaneous pedicle screws in the thoracolumbar spine. It may also be used for transpedicular biopsies or vertebral cement augmentation procedures.

This technique is contraindicated when properly aligned images of the vertebrae cannot be obtained or when the radiographic landmarks of the vertebrae cannot be adequately defined on the images. It may not be possible to obtain proper images because of obesity, severely deformed anatomy, osteopenia, retained abdominal contrast, or a poor-quality C-arm image intensifier.

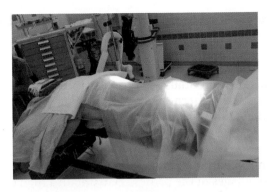

FIG. 3-1   Patient positioning on a radiolucent table.

OPERATIVE SETUP

The patient is positioned prone on a radiolucent table. Care is taken to ensure good orthogonal alignment of the patient to facilitate imaging. The bony and vital structures are padded, and the abdomen needs to be free of any compression (Fig. 3-1).

SURGICAL TECHNIQUE

Working with a C-arm technician, the surgeon fluoroscopically identifies each vertebra to be treated, and a properly aligned AP image is obtained at each vertebral level. In general, because of the sagittal profile of the spine, each vertebra requires a slightly different sagittal angulation of the C-arm to obtain a true AP view. This is especially true when imaging the S1 pedicle, where a properly angulated Ferguson view is essential for good pedicle visualization (Fig. 3-2, *A*). The C-arm is marked once the proper sagittal angle is achieved for a given vertebra to facilitate a rapid return to the proper view during the surgical procedure (Fig. 3-2, *B*).

A true AP image can be identified by the single, distinct radiopaque shadow of the upper endplate (superimposed anterior and posterior margins of the vertebral body). On a properly aligned view, the pedicles lie just inferior to the upper endplate and are sym-

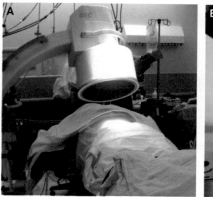
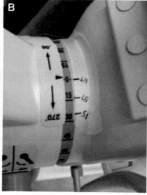

FIG. 3-2   **A,** The sagittal angulation of the C-arm must be adjusted to provide a true AP image of each vertebral level. A Ferguson-type view allows proper visualization of the S1 pedicle. **B,** A strip of tape can be used to mark the C-arm for the proper sagittal angle of each vertebra to be treated so that the correct positions can be repeated rapidly during the procedure.

metrical. To confirm that the vertebra is not rotated, the spinous process shadow must be centered between the pedicles (Fig. 3-3).

With the C-arm aligned to produce a true AP image, the surgeon identifies the trajectory to reach the pedicle by laying a K-wire over the skin of the patient's back and adjusting the position of the K-wire until it is directly in line with the center of the pedicles bilaterally (Fig. 3-4).

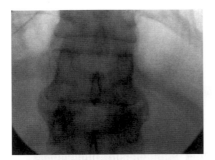

FIG. 3-3 The true AP view of a vertebra can be identified by a single radiopaque line for the superior endplate (superimposed anterior and posterior margins of the vertebral body). The pedicles lie just inferior to the upper endplate, and the spinous process is centered between the pedicle shadows.

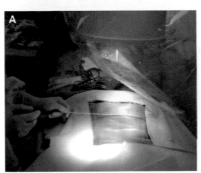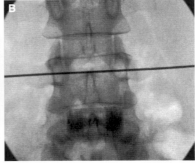

FIG. 3-4 A, A K-wire is placed on the patient's skin and aligned horizontally with the midportion of the pedicles. B, A fluoroscopic image is obtained to verify that the K-wire is centered over the midportion of the pedicle shadows.

Next, the skin is marked transversely along the K-wire positioned over the pedicles (Fig. 3-5). It is useful to mark the vertebral level and sagittal angulation of the C-arm required to obtain a true AP image. A similar process is carried out at each vertebral level to be instrumented.

A K-wire is placed on the skin and aligned vertically with the lateral border of each pedicle. Placement is confirmed with fluoroscopic imaging (Fig. 3-6).

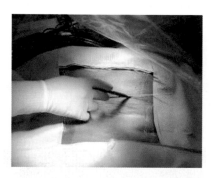

FIG. 3-5   The skin is marked along the K-wire.

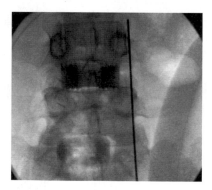

FIG. 3-6   The K-wire is placed on the patient's skin, aligned with the lateral border of the pedicles, and confirmed with fluoroscopy.

Cephalocaudal lines are marked, corresponding to the lateral borders of the pedicles to be instrumented.

Skin incisions are marked about 1 cm lateral to the line that marks the lateral border of the pedicle shadows (Fig. 3-7, *A*). Obese patients may require the skin incisions to be more lateral to accommodate the increased depth of their vertebral bodies. After the skin and fascia have been incised, the surgeon may gently dilate the tract using an index finger and then palpate the bony anatomy of the transverse process (Fig. 3-7, *B*).

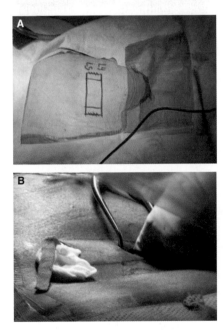

FIG. 3-7   **A,** Lines are marked along the vertically oriented K-wires. Skin incisions *(hatched lines)* are marked approximately 1 cm lateral to the lines demarcating the lateral margins of the pedicles. **B,** Digital palpation of the transverse process through the skin incision.

Jamshidi needles are inserted into the incisions and docked over the base of each of the transverse processes, which are adjacent to the lateral aspects of the facet joints (Fig. 3-8, *A*). This procedure can be carried out simultaneously by two surgeons working on either side of the spine to increase efficiency and reduce radiation exposure. The Jamshidi needles are then held in position with long Kocher clamps (Fig. 3-8, *B*). With the Jamshidi needles docked on the spine, a true AP image is obtained with the C-arm (Fig. 3-9, *A*). The goal is to place the tip of the needle directly over the mid-lateral wall of the pedicle (at the 3 o'clock position on the right and the 9 o'clock position on the left). If the needle tip is not correctly positioned, it is adjusted, and the AP image is retaken and checked until the needle tip is directly over the ideal entry site of the pedicle. The true AP view is also used to determine whether the direction of the needle is too cranial or caudal (Fig. 3-9, *B* and *C*).

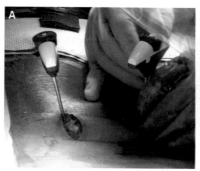 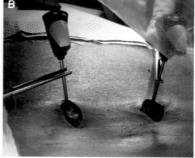

FIG. 3-8   **A,** Jamshidi needles are docked at the base of the transverse processes simultaneously by two surgeons. **B,** The needles are held with long clamps while fluoroscopic images are obtained.

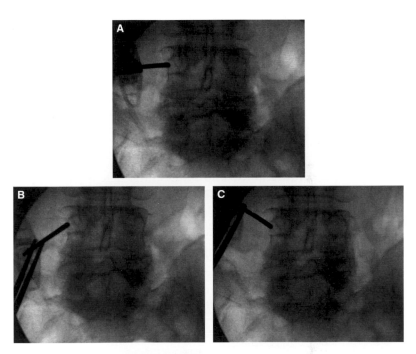

FIG. 3-9 A, In this AP image the Jamshidi needle is docked on the spine over the lateral margin of the pedicle (proper entry site to the pedicle). Notice that the shaft of the needle is parallel with the superior endplate, indicating that the needle is aligned with the pedicle axis. B, The Jamshidi needle is pointing too far cranially. C, The Jamshidi needle is pointing too far caudally.

Once the Jamshidi needle is correctly placed, it is tapped gently with a mallet to penetrate a few millimeters into the bony cortex (Fig. 3-10). Because the bony surface over the pedicle entry site is often sloping, the needle tip may slip at this point, so it is recommended that the position be checked with another true AP image before inserting the needle to the full depth of the pedicle base.

The Jamshidi needle shaft must be aligned so that it appears parallel to the upper endplate (Fig. 3-11, *A*). With the shaft in this position, the cannula will pass through the center of the pedicle. The Jamshidi needle shaft is then marked approximately 20 mm above the skin edge (Fig. 3-11, *B*) to allow the surgeon to follow the depth of penetration of the needle tip into the pedicle.

Next, holding the Jamshidi needle shaft in line with the fluoroscopic beam (parallel to the endplate on the true AP view) and with a trajectory 10 to 12 degrees of lateral-to-medial angulation, the needle is tapped to the depth of the needle mark (20 mm). At this point, the tip of the needle is approximately at the base of the pedicle (at the junction of the pedicle with the vertebral body). A true AP image is obtained to analyze the position of the needle tip relative to the pedicle shadow. The tip of the needle should be seen within the pedicle shadow one half to two thirds of the distance across the pedicle (from lateral to medial) (Fig. 3-12).

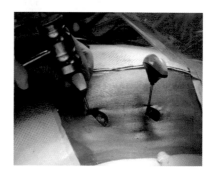

FIG. 3-10   The Jamshidi needle is tapped with a mallet to penetrate the bony cortex of the vertebra over the pedicle.

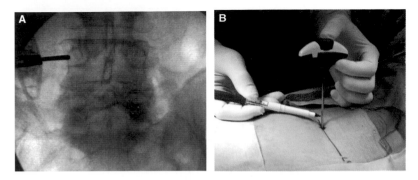

FIG. 3-11   A, The Jamshidi needle placement is confirmed, and care is taken to ensure the needle is parallel to vertebral body endplate. B, The shaft of the needle is marked 20 mm above the skin edge. This line allows the surgeon to determine the depth of needle penetration into the pedicle.

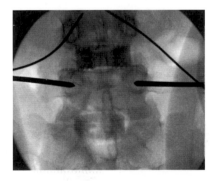

FIG. 3-12   The Jamshidi needle is within the pedicle shadow after it has been advanced 20 mm into the bone. The needle tip should be one half to two thirds of the distance across the pedicles (from lateral to medial) in a true AP view. Notice that the K-wires at the level above have a different orientation because of the lordosis of the lumbar spine.

The Jamshidi needle obturator is removed, and a blunt-tipped guidewire is introduced through the needle into the cancellous bone (Fig. 3-13). It is important for the surgeon to palpate bone at the base of the Jamshidi needle. Cancellous bone of the vertebral body feels slightly "crunchy" as the guidewire is manually advanced through it. The guidewire is then advanced 15 to 20 mm beyond the tip of the needle into the bone of the vertebral body. The Jamshidi needle shaft is removed as the guidewire is held in place. The pedicle is then tapped, and a cannulated screw is placed in the usual manner, according to the technique appropriate for the system being used.

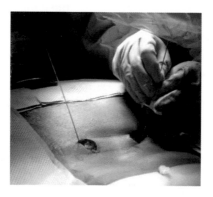

FIG. 3-13   The Jamshidi needle obturator is removed, and a blunt-tipped guidewire is introduced through the needle into the cancellous bone.

COMPLICATIONS

Complications from percutaneous pedicle cannulation are possible, resulting primarily from misplacing the Jamshidi needle or guidewire into the spinal canal or beyond the margins of the vertebral body into the abdominal or chest cavity. There are many vital structures (neurologic, vascular, and visceral) in close proximity to the vertebra that could be injured by improper placement of the needle, guidewire, or even a pedicle screw. Misplacement of the Jamshidi needle can be avoided by careful adherence to the suggested technique. The use of a sharp-tipped guidewire is discouraged, because it can migrate more easily. Maintaining constant manual control of the guidewire is crucial while cannulated instruments are being passed over it during pedicle preparation and screw insertion.

CONCLUSION

The AP fluoroscopy technique for pedicle cannulation has significant advantages and can be performed safely if all the appropriate steps are followed and close attention is given to obtaining appropriate fluoroscopic images. Many experienced MIS surgeons have found that two surgeons performing this technique simultaneously on either side of the spine provides the most efficient and accurate way to achieve pedicle cannulation, especially when working with multilevel constructs.

SURGICAL PEARLS AND PITFALLS

- *Obtain true AP views of each level to be instrumented.*

- Make sure that good images of the spinal region can be obtained before beginning surgery.

- Dock the Jamshidi needles over the 3 o'clock and 9 o'clock positions before entering them into the bony cortex.

- Obtain an AP image after cortical penetration to ensure that the needle tip has not slipped.

- Mark the needle 20 mm above the level of the skin so that the depth of needle insertion can be monitored.

- Ensure that the Jamshidi needle tip advances smoothly through the pedicle bone during needle insertion. If hard bone is encountered, the needle tip is probably too medial and has entered the facet joint, contacting the cortical surface of the superior articular process. Withdraw the needle and reposition it more laterally.

- Once the needle is in place, use a guidewire to palpate the bone at the base of the needle tip.

- Check for the distinct crunchy feel of cancellous bone.

- Maintain manual control of the guidewire while all instruments are passed over it.

BAILOUTS/ALTERNATIVE STRATEGIES

If the AP-only pedicle cannulation technique is not feasible because of poor images, open surgery should be considered. If the anatomy of the pedicle is not clear, additional fluoroscopic images, such as an owl's eye (en face) image, may prove useful for confirming the position of the pedicle.

Suggested Readings

Anand N, Baron EM, Thaiyananthan G, et al. Minimally invasive multi-level percutaneous correction and fusion for adult lumbar degenerative scoliosis: a technique and feasibility study. J Spinal Disord Tech 21:459-467, 2008.

Harris EB, Massey P, Lawrence J, Rihn J, Vaccaro A, Anderson DG. Percutaneous techniques for minimally invasive posterior lumbar fusion. Neurosurg Focus 25:E12, 2008.

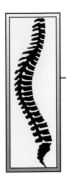

4

Owl's Eye (Magerl) Technique for Pedicle Cannulation

Michael Y. Wang

A number of techniques are available for pedicle preparation using fluoroscopic guidance. One of the earliest techniques for pedicle cannulation was described as the *owl's eye, dead reckoning,* or *Magerl*[1] technique. This method, which employs fluoroscopic imaging along the long axis of the pedicle, became accepted in Europe not only for placing percutaneous screws, but also for cement augmentation (vertebroplasty) techniques. Because of its intuitive nature and the need for only one fluoroscope, this technique was adopted rapidly during the early stages of percutaneous surgery.

INTRAOPERATIVE SETUP

As with other percutaneous techniques, the surgeon should ensure that the positioning of the operating table and patient allows for high-quality fluoroscopic imaging. Not only must the appropriate levels be imaged, but the position of the C-arm must be correct in both axial rotation and sagittal angulation. Care should be taken that the image intensifier is not obstructed by the table's platform, base, side rails, or radiopaque bolster cushions. This is particularly problematic for small-diameter C-arm devices. I prefer to use a machine with at least 32.5 inches between the image intensifier and the radiation source. Alternatively, frame-based or frameless navigation devices can be used to guide hardware placement.

SURGICAL TECHNIQUE

For bilateral pedicle screw placement, it is possible to work from only one side of the patient—typically on the side opposite the fluoroscope. Cannulation of the side across from the surgeon (the side the C-arm is on) is performed first.

The fluoroscope is aligned with the contralateral pedicle (Fig. 4-1), and care is taken that the view is truly down the pedicle. This can be assisted by examining CT and MRI axial images to ascertain the orientation and morphology of the pedicles, which can vary significantly among patients and spine levels.

Although the surgeon may elect to simply rotate the fluoroscope and alter the sagittal alignment until a desirable image is obtained, helpful information can be obtained from preoperative imaging by first aligning the sagittal plane of the fluoroscope until the upper vertebral endplate of the level of interest appears as a single line (see Chapter 3). The fluoroscope is then rotated in the axial plane to the degree of medial angulation seen on MRI or CT axial images at that level. In this manner, the precise amount of medial angulation at each level can be attained. This technique is aided by the calibration marks found on standard fluoroscopic C-arms that allow the technician to measure the degree of rotation from a strict AP alignment (Figs. 4-2 and 4-3).

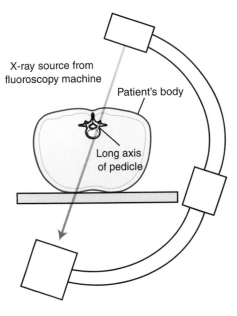

X-ray source from
fluoroscopy machine

Patient's body

Long axis
of pedicle

FIG. 4-1 Alignment of the fluoroscope for obtaining a conformal two-dimensional map of the pedicle.

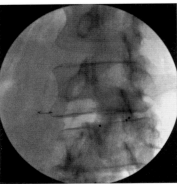

FIG. 4-2 This is an ideal view of a lumbar pedicle for the owl's eye cannulation technique. Notice the "scotty dog" figure that is used to detect pars fractures on oblique radiographs. Also notice that the alignment approximates the plane of the facet joint.

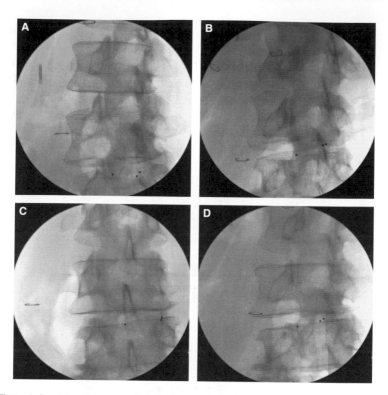

FIG. 4-3   These images do not have ideal alignment. **A** and **B**, These images have proper axial rotation but poor sagittal alignment, which is indicated by the vertebral endplates not being superimposed. In **A**, the upper vertebra is in better alignment than the lower, targeted level. **C**, This image has proper sagittal alignment, but the fluoroscope has not been rotated adequately in the axial plane. This is indicated by the spinous process being nearly in the midline and the facet joint planes being blurred. **D**, Overrotation in the axial plane. Notice that the lateral walls of the pedicle are not as clear as they are in Fig 4-2 (which is from the same patient).

Once proper images have been obtained, the incision should be made directly over the pedicle projection. Jamshidi needle placement, followed by K-wire exchange and pedicle preparation/screw placement, then proceeds as with all other techniques. During these maneuvers the cannulation is most in line with the pedicle when the instruments are superimposed over a single spot[2] (Fig. 4-4). The depth of instrument placement can be determined by periodic lateral fluoroscopic images or simply through preoperative images.

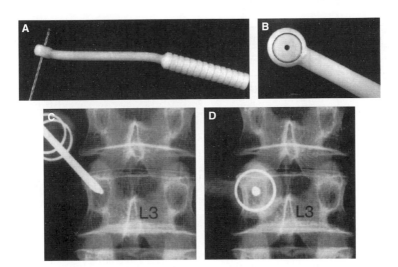

FIG. 4-4   Targeting the pedicle with a specialized instrument for confirming a dead reckoning trajectory, as described by Pennig and Brug.[2] **A** and **B**, A radiolucent holder allows targeting while keeping the surgeon's hand out of the path of the x-rays. **C**, Direct AP fluoroscopic image of the instruments being used. **D**, The radiopaque rings of the instrument are aligned and superimposed over the pedicle axis. (From Pennig D, Brug E. A target device for placement of implants in the thoracolumbar pedicles. J Bone Joint Surg Br 72:886-888, 1990. Reproduced with permission and copyright © of the British Editorial Society of Bone and Joint Surgery.)

At the S1 level the pedicle is not cylindrical. Therefore its projection appears with only the medial wall visible. Imaging for S1 requires the surgeon to first align the C-arm in the sagittal plane so that the upper sacral endplate appears as a single line. The C-arm is then rotated axially to achieve the highest resolution of the medial pedicle wall. As with the lumbar spine, this angulation can be made easier by taking measurements from preoperative axial MRI or CT scans.

COMPARISON WITH OTHER CANNULATION TECHNIQUES

Wiesner et al[3] performed a cadaveric study to compare the Magerl technique with a primarily AP technique (see Chapter 3). The authors determined that, although most misplacements were minor, the Magerl method was associated with a 13% breach rate, compared with 8% for the AP method. However, this difference was not statistically significant. Of note, the study found a high rate of medial violations with the Magerl technique. They attributed this to the more medial starting position of the pedicle screws using this method. Given the fact that the spinal canal is not visualized on the dead reckoning projection, a medial violation may go undetected. Therefore surgeons using this method should exercise great care to start the cannulation process in a lateral position, at the junction of the transverse process and facet joint.

The study also found that it was easier to handle the fluoroscope with the AP technique, an experience that I share, because this method does not require realigning the fluoroscope twice for each level, thus increasing the amount of C-arm manipulation. Although the owl's eye method requires substantially fewer images to be taken than the biplanar method, it likely results in more radiation exposure than AP targeting.

CONCLUSION

The owl's eye technique is a highly intuitive method for safe percutaneous pedicle cannulation. It may be a useful technique when AP imaging proves difficult because image guidance or biplanar fluoroscopy is not available. The technique is easily adopted and requires a minimum of specialized equipment.

SURGICAL PEARLS AND PITFALLS

- Care must be taken to ensure proper alignment of the fluoroscope so that the upper vertebral endplate appears as a single line and the pedicle is a perfect oval (except at S1).

- When placing either a Jamshidi needle or a K-wire, the instrument should appear as a single dot on the fluoroscopic image.

- The depth of penetration can be measured preoperatively or with a lateral fluoroscopic image.

- Record the degrees of angulation in the sagittal and axial planes for each side and level of the spine in case it becomes necessary to return the fluoroscope to a previous side or level.

- Medial violations are more likely to occur with the owl's eye method. Entering the pedicle at the lateral facet joint can help reduce this problem.

References

1. Magerl F. Verletzungen der Brust- und Lendenwirbelsaule. Langenbecks Arch Chir 352:428-433, 1980.
2. Pennig D, Brug E. A target device for placement of implants in the thoracolumbar pedicles. J Bone Joint Surg Br 72:886-888, 1990.
3. Wiesner L, Kothe R, Ruther W. Anatomic evaluation of two different techniques for the percutaneous insertion of pedicle screws in the lumbar spine. Spine 24:1599-1603, 1999.

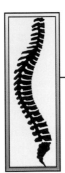

5

Mini-Open Technique for Pedicle Cannulation, TLIF, and Decompression

Jason S. Taub, Sanjay S. Dhall,
Praveen V. Mummaneni

I n 1968 Wiltse et al[1] first described the paraspinal sacrospinalis muscle-splitting approach to the lumbar spine. This approach is best suited for one-level fusions in patients with spondylolisthesis. In the sagittal plane, the lumbar musculature was dissected in a manner that decreased bleeding and provided a more direct approach to the transverse processes and pedicles. Unlike the traditional midline incision, it was also thought to decrease postoperative pain and avoid disruption of the supraspinous and interspinous ligaments.[2] These principles have been incorporated into the mini-open technique for posterior spinal instrumentation. This chapter describes the basic mini-open technique of pedicle cannulation for screw placement using an expandable tube, as well as our technique for mini-open transforaminal lumbar interbody fusion (TLIF).

INDICATIONS AND CONTRAINDICATIONS

The mini-open technique using an expandable tubular retractor provides an alternative to the standard open surgical technique of pedicle screw insertion. Spinal instability or deformity resulting from scoliosis, spondylolisthesis, trauma, tumors, or infections, as well as low back pain and disc disease, can be treated using the mini-open technique.[3] The indications for surgery summarized in the lumbar fusion guidelines (Box 5-1) should be considered before offering patients either mini-open or open spinal fusion surgery.[4] In patients who have undergone midline open operations, a paramedian mini-open approach avoids reopening the old incision, decreasing the incidence of durotomy. Decreased blood loss and muscle trauma and shorter hospital stays have been associated with transforaminal lumbar interbody fusion (TLIF) procedures using the mini-open approach.[2] In high-risk surgical patients (specifically, elderly, obese, and immunocompromised patients), procedures with less blood loss are often preferred.

Relative contraindications to the mini-open approach using an expandable tubular retractor include fusions of three or more segments (the retractors usually only expand to two levels), exposures deeper than 8 cm (the maximum retractor depth), high-grade spondylolisthesis, and deformity requiring osteotomies or multilevel reduction (see Box 5-1). In addition, patients with distorted anatomic landmarks for pedicle fixation (that is, those with prior posterolateral fusions) are not ideal candidates for a mini-open technique.

Box 5-1
Relative Indications and Contraindications for Mini-Open Lumbar Fusion

Relative Indications

Spondylolisthesis (usually grade I or II)

Degenerative disc disease causing discogenic low back pain (one or two levels)

Recurrent lumbar disc herniation with significant mechanical back pain

Postdiscectomy collapse with neural foraminal stenosis and radiculopathy

Third time (or more) of recurrent lumbar disc herniation with radiculopathy (with or without back pain)

Pseudarthrosis

Postlaminectomy kyphosis

Relative Contraindications

High-grade spondylolisthesis (grade III or IV)

Deformity cases requiring osteotomies or reduction maneuvers

Three or more levels of spinal disease requiring treatment

One-level disc disease causing radiculopathy without symptoms of mechanical low back pain or instability

Severe osteoporosis

More than 8 cm of tissue depth

Altered posterolateral anatomic landmarks

Adapted from Lu DC, Mummaneni PV. Mini-open approaches. In Perez-Cruet MJ, Pimenta L, Beisse R, eds. Minimally Invasive Spine Fusion: Techniques and Operative Nuances. St Louis: Quality Medical Publishing, 2011.

PREOPERATIVE PLANNING
History and Physical Examination

The surgeon should assess the detailed history and perform a thorough physical examination for evidence of neurologic compromise resulting from mechanical instability or neural compression. Motor strength, sensory deficits, reflexes, range of motion, and long tract signs should be carefully documented.

Radiographic Workup

Recognizing any degree of scoliosis or kyphosis is important for preoperative planning. Neurogenic claudication, low back pain, and radicular symptoms should be investigated with radiographic images. Plain AP and lateral lumbar films may show spondylolisthesis or traumatic fractures; however, MRI is better for revealing neural compression, disc herniation, and other soft tissue pathology (Fig. 5-1). Likewise, lateral flexion and extension films (dy-

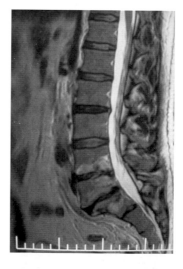

FIG. 5-1   This MRI image shows degenerative spondylosis at L4-5 and L5-S1.

namic radiographs) help the examination of pathologic motion segments in the lumbar region. In patients with osteoporosis or an underlying malignancy, a CT scan of the lumbar spine may assist in further assessment of bone quality. Of particular importance is the depth of tissue from the skin surface to the spine (measured with axial CT or MRI), which should be determined to ensure the applicability of the mini-open approach. Soft tissue measurements of 8 cm or more may be a relative contraindication.

OPERATIVE SETUP

The patient is positioned prone on a Jackson table with supportive chest and pelvic pads. Be careful when using an open-bottom operating table with obese patients, because the weight of their pannus can result in hyperlordosis. For such patients we often use a Wilson frame on a Jackson table to provide more support for the pannus (Fig. 5-2). We also prefer to use a Jackson table with a Wilson frame for patients with severe lumbar stenosis in addition to spondylolisthesis. During the interlaminar decompression, we

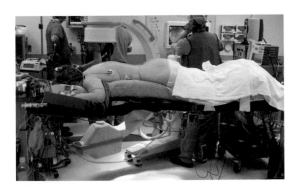

FIG. 5-2   The patient is positioned prone on a Jackson table with a Wilson frame in a lordotic position. Arms are abducted to 90 degrees at the shoulders and elbows to enhance fluoroscopic imaging.

raise, or "crank up," the Wilson frame to splay the lamina apart, which tenses the ligamentum flavum and makes decompression easier. After the decompression, we lower ("crank down") the Wilson frame into a lordotic position. We fixate the rods to the screw heads after the frame is in lordosis to avoid fixing the patient in a flat-back position. The arms are typically abducted at the shoulders to avoid interference with fluoroscopy. Perioperative antibiotics are given before the skin is incised. We typically use intraoperative electromyography (EMG) during decompression and/or instrumentation, and we check screw stimulation thresholds with EMG to help avoid medial breaches of the pedicle screws.

SURGICAL TECHNIQUE
Initial Incision and Placement of Dilators and Tubular Retractor

Fluoroscopy is used to identify and mark the skin overlying the appropriate level for the incision location. Specifically, on the AP view, we mark the patient's skin with the superimposed position of the pedicles bordering the intended level or levels of fusion. The incision extends from the outside margins of the pedicle locations, approximately 3 to 4 cm laterally to midline, which allows the Wiltse paraspinal muscle-splitting approach to be performed[5] (Fig. 5-3). After incising the skin and fascia, a plane is developed between the multifidus and longissimus muscles, and this pathway to the spine is progressively enlarged with sequential dilator tubes. An expandable tubular retractor can then be positioned. The inner dilators are easily removed (Fig. 5-4). A snake arm attached from the side of the operating table to the expandable tubular retractor adds stability and allows angulation.

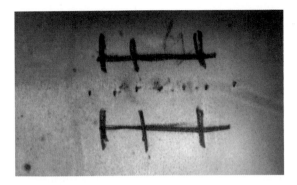

FIG. 5-3 The *dotted line* represents the midline, with bilateral incisions marked over the pedicles laterally. In this case, a two-level mini-open TLIF is planned.

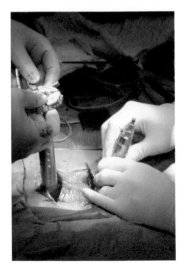

FIG. 5-4 Sequentially enlarging dilator tubes are inserted over one another *(right)*, with an expandable tubular retractor (Pipeline, DePuy Spine, Raynham, MA) positioned over the fifth dilator *(left)*.

Pedicle Cannulation

Using Bovie electrocautery and dissecting curettes, the lateral facet complex, transverse processes, pars interarticularis, and pedicle are identified and exposed. Care should be taken not to injure the facet above the intended fusion site when exposing the superior transverse process and superior pedicle screw entry site. The pedicle screw entry point (the junction of the midpoint of the lumbar transverse process with the lateral aspect of the superior articulating facet) is decorticated with a high-speed drill. A gearshift is used to navigate down the pedicle into the vertebral body (similar to a standard open approach). After the pedicle is probed and tapped, a small amount of a flowable hemostatic agent is placed in the pedicle hole (Fig. 5-5). If necessary, a foraminotomy for nerve root decompression can be performed, and a hemilaminectomy can be achieved with medial angulation of the tubular retractor. This technique is repeated for any additional levels of instrumentation.[1,5]

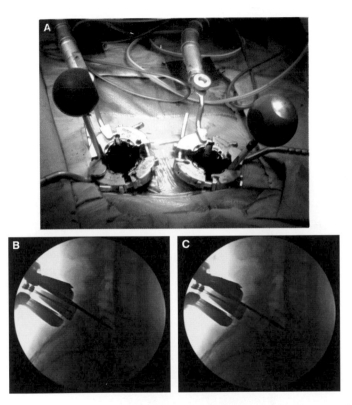

FIG. 5-5   A, Gearshifts are placed into the pedicles through the expandable tubular retractors. B, Lateral fluoroscopic view of the gearshift through the pedicle. C, The tap is inserted through the pedicle before final screw placement.

Transforaminal Lumbar Interbody Fusion

If a TLIF is to be performed, the surgeon first cannulates the pedicles adjacent to the intended TLIF disc space. The pedicle screws are not placed until the interbody space is prepared and the TLIF cage is inserted; otherwise, the pedicle screw heads may impede access to the disc space. After the pedicle screw pathways have been created, small pedicle markers can be placed in the prepared

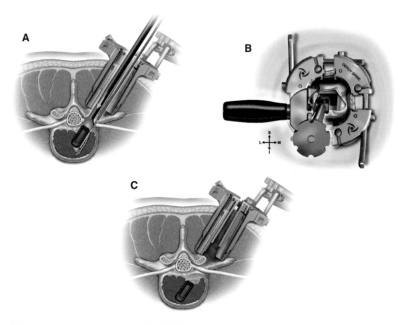

FIG. 5-6   A, Placement of a TLIF cage using a mini-open approach with an expandable retractor. B, View through an expandable retractor while placing a TLIF cage into the disc space. C, The cage is in position with bone graft in the cage and surrounding it. (Images © DePuy Spine, Inc. 2010. All rights reserved. Used with permission.)

bony holes. These markers provide anatomic visual cues and help the surgeon avoid violating the pedicles with the drill.

At this point a facetectomy and foraminotomy are performed with a drill or small chisel and mallet to expose the disc space, which is just above the lower pedicle screw cannulation hole. The disc is incised with a long-handled scalpel and removed with endplate shavers, pituitary rongeurs, and curettes. Care should be taken to remove the cartilaginous interbody endplates without injuring the bony vertebral body endplates both above and below the disc space. Interbody trials are used to serially dilate the interbody space. An appropriate cage is then selected based on the trial that has a secure fit, and it is implanted into the disc space (Fig. 5-6). Subsequently, the pedicle markers are removed and the pedicle screws are placed.

Decompression of the Neural Elements

After the TLIF has been completed, if a spinal canal decompression is needed, it can be performed by angling the expandable tube medially onto the hemilamina. An ipsilateral hemilaminectomy can then be performed using a high-speed drill and small bone punches and curettes. By angling the tube even more, the contralateral lamina can also be visualized and thinned ventrally with a drill to increase the canal diameter. The ligamentum flavum may be removed with curettes after the bony work has been done. We remove the ligamentum flavum after all drill work is finished to reduce the risk of spinal fluid leakage.

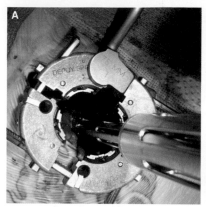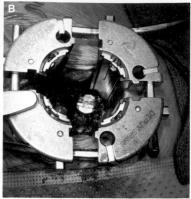

FIG. 5-7   **A,** The surgeon's view of the pedicle screw insertion through an expandable tubular retractor. **B,** The pedicle screw is in position.

Placement of Pedicle Screws

An appropriate-size pedicle screw is inserted at each level (Fig. 5-7). Screw stimulation with EMG monitoring is performed to help verify that there are no medial screw breaches. In general, screw stimulation thresholds of 5 mAmp or lower should alert the surgeon to a potential medial pedicle wall breach.

Placement of Bone Graft and Rods

The bony facet surface is decorticated. Bone graft is placed over the transverse process and may be packed into the facet joint. Next, a measured rod is secured to the pedicle screw heads with locking caps (Fig. 5-8).

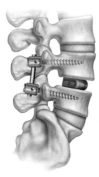

FIG. 5-8 A completed TLIF construct in the lumbar spine, including the cage packed with autograft and pedicle screw–rod fixation. (Image © DePuy Spine, Inc. 2010. All rights reserved. Used with permission.)

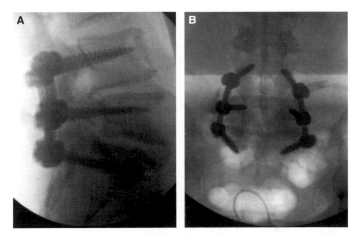

FIG. 5-9 A, Lateral fluoroscopy showing the pedicle screw and rod construct. B, AP view of the same construct.

Closure

The wound is irrigated with antibiotic solution and hemostasis is confirmed. The retractor tube is removed, and the fascia and skin are closed in a layered fashion. If applicable, the same steps are followed for the contralateral side. We recommend using fluoroscopy to verify the screw position before removing the sterile drapes (Fig. 5-9).

COMPLICATIONS

Potential complications that can occur during a mini-open procedure include instrument malposition and dural injury. Because of the limited exposure and reduced working space, appropriate pedicle screw placement can be difficult and requires excellent working knowledge of the anatomy seen through the tubular retractor. AP and lateral fluoroscopy can help locate the pedicle screw entry points and assist with anatomic reference points. Before the screw is placed, a small, ball-tipped feeler probe is used to palpate the inside walls of the pedicle to assess any wall violations. If a pedicle wall breach is identified, then an alternative trajectory can be found with fluoroscopy.

To minimize the potential for dural tears, we prefer to prepare and tap the pedicle screw entry points before exposing the nerve roots or thecal sac. Cerebrospinal fluid leaks can be difficult to repair when using a limited approach. However, if a leak occurs, we attempt to close the dural defect primarily using a small needle driver and running dural suture. If this is not possible, then we approximate the dural edges with a suture. A small piece of dural substitute and fibrin glue are applied to the region to create a seal. If necessary, a lumbar drain may be placed for additional cerebrospinal fluid diversion. One advantage of the smaller opening is a decreased space for potential pseudomeningocele formation.

CONCLUSION

The mini-open technique allows pedicle preparation in a manner similar to the open surgical approach. A TLIF may also be performed using a tubular retractor system.

SURGICAL PEARLS AND PITFALLS

- For obese patients, make the initial incision farther from midline (more lateral) to allow for an adequate lateral-to-medial pedicle trajectory.

- Avoid using a K-wire before inserting the dilator tube during a mini-open approach, because it may result in an unintended durotomy.

- Take the time to identify initial landmarks with fluoroscopy before bony decompression or instrumentation. Because of the limited visualization provided by tubular retractors, the lamina may be mistaken for the transverse process, leading to attempted placement of the pedicle screw at the lamina/spinous process junction instead of at the transverse process/facet junction. Fluoroscopy helps minimize such errors.

- To minimize dural injury, interbody fusion or bony decompression is performed after preparing pedicle entry sites, but before screw placement.

BAILOUTS/ALTERNATIVE STRATEGIES

The need to convert from a mini-open approach to a traditional large midline open procedure is very rare in our experience. Preoperative evaluation is essential to determine the appropriate procedure for each patient and will help avoid this conversion.

References

1. Wiltse LL, Bateman G, Hutchinson RH, et al. The paraspinal sacro-spinalis-splitting approach to the lumbar spine. J Bone Joint Surg Am 50:919-926, 1968.
2. Dhall SS, Wang MY, Mummaneni PV. Clinical and radiographic comparison of mini-open transforaminal lumbar interbody fusion with open transforaminal lumbar interbody fusion in 42 patients with long-term follow-up. J Neurosurg Spine 9:560-565, 2008.
3. Lu DC, Dhall SS, Mummaneni PV. Mini-open removal of extradural foraminal tumors of the lumbar spine. J Neurosurg Spine 10:46-50, 2009.
4. Resnick DK, Choudhri TF, Dailey AT, Groff MW, Khoo L, Matz PG, Mummaneni P, et al. Guidelines for the performance of fusion procedures for degenerative disease of the lumbar spine. Part 12: pedicle screw fixation as an adjunct to posterolateral fusion for low-back pain. J Neurosurg Spine 2:700-706, 2005.
5. Mummaneni PV, Rodts GE Jr. The mini-open transforaminal lumbar interbody fusion. Neurosurgery 57(4 Suppl):256-261; discussion 256-261, 2005.

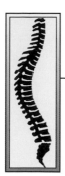

6

Minimally Invasive Approaches for Lateral Lumbar Interbody Fusion

Kelley E. Banagan, Steven C. Ludwig

L umbar fusion is indicated in a variety of clinical scenarios, including the management of degenerative, neoplastic, developmental, infectious, and traumatic conditions of the spine. Minimally invasive fusion techniques have evolved to reduce soft tissue collateral damage associated with the surgical approach. The basic tenet of these novel techniques is to achieve the same surgical goals as open procedures, but with reduced morbidity, thus hastening postoperative recovery.

One such minimally invasive technique is the direct lateral interbody approach. This approach has been presented as a safe and reproducible technique for reconstructing sagittal and coronal imbalance, indirectly decompressing the neural elements, and acting as a medium to introduce the biologic agents for fusion. Using specially designed expandable retractors, a surgical working zone is created with the assistance of intraoperative fluoroscopy. The procedure can often be performed without the assistance of an exposure surgeon. It is typically used for the lumbar spine from L1 through L5. Proponents of this technique are beginning to use the approach for the thoracic spine. Advantages of this technique over other minimally invasive surgical techniques, such as transforaminal lumbar interbody fusion or posterior lumbar interbody fusion, are a more thorough discectomy, greater correction of deformity, and the placement of a larger interbody cage device that delivers the biologic agent.

PATIENT POSITIONING

Patient positioning is important for both visualization and the ease with which the procedure can be performed. The direct lateral interbody approach is performed with the patient in the lateral decubitus position, with a lateral bolster placed to open the interval between the twelfth rib and the iliac crest. This can be accomplished with the patient on an OSI table (Mizuho OSI, Union City, CA), using an inflatable 3 L saline infusion bag as the bolster to flex the spine. Alternatively, placing the patient on a regular radiolucent table and reverse flexing it so that the break in the table is at the level of the iliac crest also creates the surgical working zone. When using a standard operative table, the patient is taped to the table with one piece of tape across the chest beneath the arms, one piece across the hips to pull the iliac crest inferiorly, and one piece across the lower limbs (Fig. 6-1). The patient should be positioned with the hips and knees slightly flexed to relax the psoas musculature.

Patient positioning is of paramount importance when the technique is being used to address pathologic conditions at the L4-5 level. This disc space can be difficult to access because of its position relative to the iliac crest; maximizing the break in the table and following the suggested taping technique improves access (Fig. 6-2). All bony prominences are adequately padded; the head and neck are propped; if needed, a nasogastric tube is placed; and appropriate antibiotics are administered before incision.

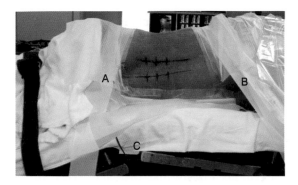

FIG. 6-1 Patient positioning on the operating table. A piece of tape is placed over the iliac crest (*A*), to pull it posteriorly, and another piece is placed across the chest (*B*) to place traction on the rib cage cranially. Then the table is reverse flexed so that the break is at the iliac crest (*C*).

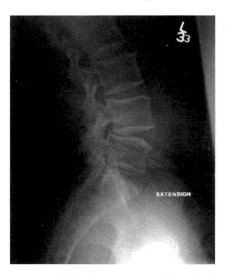

FIG. 6-2 The position of the iliac crest is evaluated relative to the disc.

Prone Positioning

Prone positioning is an alternative to lateral positioning and offers the advantage of avoiding major repositioning if a prone approach is needed for a concurrent procedure. Lumbar interbody fusion performed with the patient prone is designed to avoid mobilization of the great vessels and to preserve the posterior anatomy of the stabilizing structures. Furthermore, it allows direct visualization and protection of the nerves and provides an alternative for revision procedures. However, when approaching the spine laterally while the patient is positioned prone, the surgeon should consider the following:

- The bed rail should be positioned so that it does not encumber the approach (particularly if the patient has settled ventrally into the table).
- The approach should still be directly lateral, because it is easier to deviate more ventrally, which tends to result in docking on the anterior aspect of the vertebral body.
- The surgeon may become easily fatigued from the unusual approach, but this can be mitigated by using a stool with adjustable height and armrests.

SURGICAL TECHNIQUE

Approach and Dissection

Fluoroscopy is used to identify the level of interest, and an incision is made in the flank overlying the psoas musculature and the disc space. True AP and lateral fluoroscopic views are obtained, and the anterior third of the disc space and the anterior and posterior limits of the vertebral bodies are localized. The position of the patient on the table should be adjusted accordingly. Accurate visualization of the disc space and appropriate fluoroscopic adjustments are made before dissection. A one-incision technique has become popular, because it allows direct visualization. Blunt dissection is then performed through the external and internal oblique musculature and the transversalis.

Transpsoas Technique Versus Posterior Sweep

The transpsoas technique requires sequential dilation of the anterior third of the psoas musculature. The lumbar plexus, composed of the anterior rami of the L1, L2, and L3 nerve roots and part of the L4 anterior ramus, is located within the substance of the psoas muscle on the posterior abdominal wall. The original authors of the technique recommend remaining in the anterior third of the muscle to avoid potential damage to the plexus and the genitofemoral nerve[1] (Fig. 6-3, *A*). However, recent anatomic and clinical studies have shown that the plexus is vulnerable to injury even in the anterior third of the psoas musculature.[2]

To avoid iatrogenic neural injuries, we recommend that dissection begin in a plane on the anterior border of the psoas muscle. The entire psoas muscle is then retracted posteriorly off the disc space with a Cobb elevator. This technique is performed with direct visualization of the psoas muscle to identify and protect any traversing nerve roots of the plexus (Fig. 6-3, *B*). Once the psoas muscle has been mobilized, sequential dilators are inserted over the guidewire at the level of the targeted disc space.

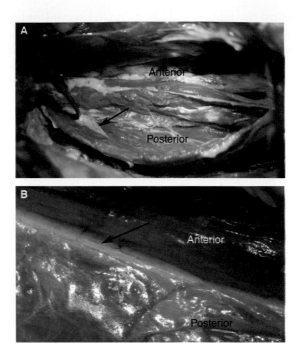

FIG. 6-3   **A,** Psoas muscle anatomy. Perforating branches of the lumbar plexus course throughout the psoas muscle *(arrow).* **B,** The genitofemoral nerve overlies the psoas musculature *(arrow).*

Neuromonitoring

Some authors[1] have described the use of a specialized neuromonitoring device during the sequential dilation of the psoas muscle when performing the transpsoas approach. To date, no published data have supported using this device, validated its accuracy, or shown its effectiveness in preventing injury to the plexus. We advocate standard techniques of intraoperative neuromonitoring with either spontaneous or triggered electromyographic recording from the lower extremity. We do not think it is necessary for surgeons to use commercially available neuromonitoring devices.

Discectomy

Once the psoas muscle has been swept posteriorly, the vertebral bodies and respective disc spaces are easily identified (Fig. 6-4, *A*), and thorough discectomy is performed (Fig. 6-4, *B*). An annulotomy is made in a box-cut fashion. A Cobb elevator can be used to release the anulus to the contralateral side. It is important to avoid violation of the bony endplates. Fluoroscopy is valuable for guiding the surgeon, with placement of the Cobb elevator down the vertebral endplate. Commercially available curettes, rasps, bone rongeurs, and Kerrison rongeurs allow a thorough discectomy. Sequential dilators allow maximal coronal and sagittal plane corrections. Once appropriate discectomy, release, and dilations have been performed, the interbody device is placed. As a general rule, the device used should be the largest that the space can accommodate.

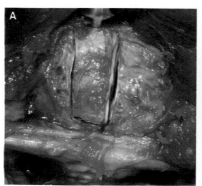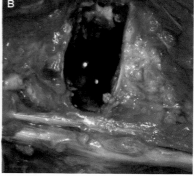

FIG. 6-4   **A,** The disc spaces are identified after the psoas muscle is swept posteriorly. **B,** The discectomy is completed.

SURGICAL CONSIDERATIONS
Convex Versus Concave Approaches for Deformity Correction

The importance of preoperative planning is best illustrated when using the direct lateral approach and interbody fusion to correct adult degenerative scoliosis. Careful consideration is essential for determining which side of the curve will be addressed (Fig. 6-5). On the convexity of the curve, the disc spaces are wider and easier to access, but the surgical approach and exposure need to be greater to allow visualization of the necessary levels. On the concavity of the curve, the disc spaces are smaller and more difficult to access, but the approach is smaller. Sequential wanding of the expandable retractor allows a discectomy to be performed using a

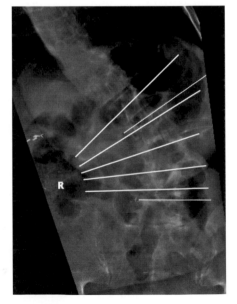

FIG. 6-5   Differences between the convex and the concave sides of a scoliotic curve.

centralized approach. If addressing the concavity of the curve, discectomies should be performed first at the proximal and distal extents of the curve. Working sequentially from the outer portion of the curve toward the apical region of the curve maximizes the correction of the spinal deformity.

Instrumentation to Maintain Stability

After lateral interbody fusion is completed, the need for instrumentation to maintain stability is considered. With a single-level fusion, the choices include placing a stand-alone interbody cage, lateral plating, or a posterior percutaneous pedicle or facet screw. The surgeon should use his or her discretion to implement the instrumentation that he or she is most comfortable with applying, understanding that all are potentially viable options. However, in cases of fusion at multiple levels for deformity correction, we favor posterior minimally invasive pedicle screws for final correction and stability.

COMPLICATIONS

The surgeon must be aware of surrounding anatomy to avoid potential complications. The conus medullaris, cauda equina, and nerve roots lie posterior to the disc space. Inadvertent posterior placement of an interbody cage places these structures at risk. Lumbar plexus neurapraxia and hip flexor weakness have been reported postoperatively. Damage to the genitofemoral nerve has also been reported, with resultant groin and thigh paresthesias.

Vascular injuries can occur with dissection anterior to the disc space. Structures at risk include the aorta and the vena cava. Additionally, with aggressive sweeping of the retractor or expansion of the retractor superiorly or inferiorly, the lumbar segmental vessels can be damaged. Injury to any of these structures can result in uncontrollable blood loss.

When closing the fascial and muscle layers, care must be taken to avoid the formation of a hernia. Our current protocol is to close the external oblique fascia in an interrupted fashion, followed by subcutaneous and cutaneous layered closure. No other fascial envelopes or muscle layers are closed.

POSTOPERATIVE CARE

At the close of the procedure, an injection of methylprednisolone acetate (Depo-Medrol) may be administered at the surgical site to treat psoas irritation and pain postoperatively. Patients are advanced to a regular diet as tolerated and are maintained on a standard course of postoperative antibiotics for 24 hours. Patients are encouraged to ambulate and to work with physical and occupational therapists. Active and passive range of motion exercises of the lower extremities, as well as stretching and isometric strengthening of the lower extremity muscles, are encouraged for the first 6 weeks after the procedure. Nonimpact aerobic conditioning is implemented for the first 6 weeks to improve the patient's endurance and overall sense of well-being.

CONCLUSION

The direct lateral interbody fusion approach is a safe and reproducible technique for reconstructing sagittal and coronal imbalance, indirectly decompressing the neural elements, and introducing a cage with biologic agents for fusion. The technique can be performed in a minimally invasive fashion for a variety of spinal disorders, including degenerative, traumatic, infectious, and deformative. A thorough understanding of the anatomic constraints and careful preparation of the surgical working zone are essential for a successful outcome.

SURGICAL PEARLS AND PITFALLS

- The transpsoas approach should be used with caution because of its proximity to the lumbosacral plexus. An alternative is to sweep the psoas muscle posteriorly before discectomy and fusion.

- Approach L4-5 with caution, because high rates of neural injury have been reported with this approach.

- When choosing between the convexity and the concavity of a scoliosis curve for the approach, entry is often best through the side that gives better access to the ends of the curve, which is typically the side that allows entry into L4-5 over the iliac crest.

- Interbody release and cage placement should start with the ends, and the apex should be managed last.

- Releasing the contralateral anulus with a Cobb elevator is essential for placing an interbody graft of adequate height.

Acknowledgment

We thank senior editor and writer Dori Kelly, MA, for her invaluable assistance in the preparation of the manuscript and figures for this chapter.

References

1. Ozgur BM, Aryan HE, Pimenta L, et al. Extreme lateral interbody fusion (XLIF): a novel surgical technique for anterior lumbar interbody fusion. Spine J 6:435-443, 2006.
2. Knight RQ, Schwaegler P, Hanscom D, et al. Direct lateral lumbar interbody fusion for degenerative conditions: early complication profile. J Spinal Disord Tech 22:34-37, 2009.

Suggested Reading

Tormenti MJ, Maserati MB, Bonfield CM, et al. Complications and radiographic correction in adult scoliosis following combined transpsoas extreme lateral interbody fusion and posterior pedicle screw instrumentation. Neurosurg Focus 28:E7, 2010.

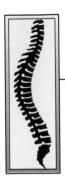

7

Multilevel Minimally Invasive Rod Passage Techniques

Steven C. Ludwig, Michael Y. Wang, Praveen V. Mummaneni

Minimally invasive spine fixation is accomplished with a set of surgical techniques and principles that emphasize soft-tissue preservation while maintaining the established foundations of fixation. Some of the established advantages of minimally invasive spine surgery are that it results in less muscle damage, less paraspinal muscle denervation, less perioperative blood loss, lower infection rates, shorter hospital stays, and less time off from work.

During the past several years, with the introduction of new screw technologies, interest has grown in performing minimally invasive procedures for more complex conditions of the thoracolumbar spine. Because the goals of surgery cannot be compromised, complex spinal conditions often require complex multilevel solutions. For this chapter, we define multilevel procedures as those requiring a rod to be passed through at least four screws.

INDICATIONS AND CONTRAINDICATIONS

Multilevel, minimally invasive procedures are being used by spine surgeons for a variety of complex spinal conditions, both adult and pediatric. The number of levels for which a rod can be applied using a minimally invasive thoracolumbar procedure seems almost unlimited. Multilevel constructs can be used to treat the following conditions:

- Traumatic thoracolumbar injury: Unstable burst fractures, flexion-distraction injuries, extension-distraction injuries, fracture-dislocations, and lumbopelvic fixation for unstable sacral fractures
- Deformity: Adult and pediatric idiopathic scoliosis, adult degenerative scoliosis, posttraumatic deformities, and kyphosis, as well as topping off procedures to prevent adjacent segment kyphosis and/or fracture
- Infection: Postinfectious deformities and posterior stabilization after osteomyelitis and/or anterior debridement of vertebral discitis
- Tumor: Posterior stabilization of pathologic fractures secondary to metastatic spinal disease and posterior stabilization after anterior excision of spinal lesions

An absolute contraindication to multilevel rod passage through a minimally invasive incision is an inability to visualize the pedicle anatomy using radiographic imaging. Without visualization, pedicle screws and their extensions cannot be placed accurately. Relative contraindications include systemic infection and severe osteoporosis. Although there have been concerns that the passage of longer or curved rods may be difficult, if the pedicle screws are placed properly and basic technical principles are followed, this step is typically straightforward.

PREOPERATIVE PLANNING

Careful preoperative planning is of paramount importance for safe and accurate rod placement. Any significant disparity between adjacent pedicle screw saddles may make rod-screw connection difficult. In addition, because of the mechanical advantages afforded by modern minimally invasive systems, screw pullout becomes a legitimate concern if too great a force is applied to the screws during rod attachment. Proper planning of screw entry points and attention to screw head depths can help prevent these problems. As with open surgery, multiple rod passages may be needed to bend the rods properly for complex or multiplane deformities. However, rod passage itself is surprisingly easy for multilevel procedures.

SURGICAL TECHNIQUE

After spine surgeons have mastered minimally invasive fixation techniques for one- and two-level spinal conditions, attempting multilevel procedures should be considered.

Rod Passage

After the surgeon has successfully placed the percutaneous pedicle screws, the rod length should be measured or estimated, and then it must be contoured before passage. For rod passage, we advocate a two-handed technique to obtain proper sensory feedback (Fig. 7-1). With the two-handed technique, the surgeon's dominant hand is on the rod holder, and the contralateral hand manipulates the screw extensions. The dominant hand is aimed toward the contralateral hand. By simultaneously pushing the rod holder and carefully rotating and derotating the screw extensions, accurate rod placement can be achieved in multilevel constructs.

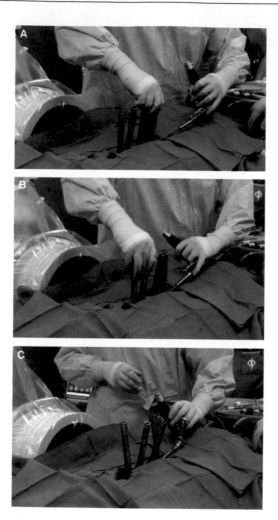

FIG. 7-1   A, Insertion of a rod attached to a specialized holder with a ratchet for axial rotation during and after insertion. B, The rod has been passed through all of the screw extensions. C, The rod is axially rotated, as can be seen by the position of the rod holder.

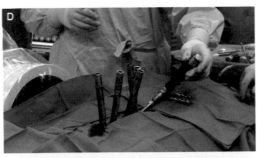

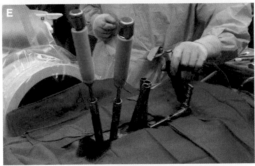

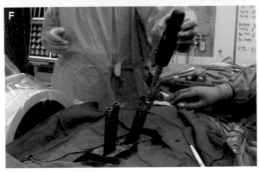

FIG. 7-1, cont'd D, The rod has now been rotated 180 degrees. Notice the change in alignment of the screw extensions. E, Set screws are used to fix the screws to the rod. F, In its ideal final position, the rod may not fully engage the screw saddles. A specialized tool moves the rod into the screw saddles while manipulating the spine into a more ideal position.

There are several methods for determining whether a rod has been placed accurately through the screw extensions, as follows:

- If a screw extension can be turned 360 degrees after rod passage, then the rod has been placed outside the screw extension. If the screw extension is blocked from turning, rod placement has been achieved through it.
- The rod can be seen directly in the screw extensions with proper lighting and suction.
- Proper passage through a screw extension may also be determined by placing a screwdriver into the extension and receiving tactile feedback of rod movements.

A curved rod is easier to guide through the soft tissues to capture the pedicle screw saddles. Fig. 7-2 shows a double-curved rod being passed through the extensions of screws that have been placed in the thoracolumbar junction and in the lumbar spine. The curves

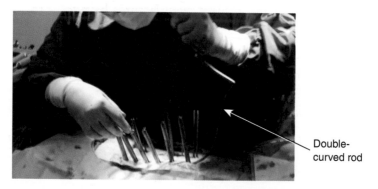

Double-curved rod

FIG. 7-2   A double-curved rod is passed through the extensions of screws that have been placed in the thoracolumbar junction and lumbar spine. The curves of the rod are intended to work with the kyphosis and lordosis of these two spinal sections, respectively.

of the rod are intended to work with the kyphosis and lordosis of these two spinal sections, respectively. The rod is turned along its long axis to guide it medially or laterally.

When introducing the rod into the first screw extension, the surgeon should drive the tip of the rod toward the screw head in a way to ensure that the rod is placed in the subfascial zone. If rod placement seems difficult, the surgeon should consider that inadvertent rod passage above the fascia might be diverting the rod into the wrong trajectory. This typically is verified if the rod appears in a too posterior position on lateral fluoroscopy. To prevent incorrect passage of the rod, care should be taken to minimize cutting the fascia too much either superiorly or inferiorly before placing pedicle screws.

Rod Length Determination and Contouring

Determining the correct rod length is often difficult with multilevel constructs. Most implant manufactures have tools to facilitate this process, but multiple checks should be conducted to ensure the proper length. An overall evaluation of the distance from the first screw extension through the last can help determine the accuracy of the chosen rod length. Often, before contouring, the surgeon may be able to pass the rod externally through all of the screw extensions to verify the length. For multilevel constructs, it is important to choose a rod length that exceeds the true distance from the first through last screw extension. Doing so allows for the increased length required for contouring.

Proper rod contouring is a key element of facilitating rod passage with multilevel thoracolumbar constructs. It is an art that can be mastered with experience. Knowledge of the appropriate amounts of thoracic kyphosis and lumbar lordosis is also essential for successful contouring. Additionally, the patient's underlying condition and radiographic studies need to be scrutinized when building the final implant construct. This is critical for percutaneous surgery, because the entire assembly occurs beneath the soft tissue envelope, and it is not possible to directly visualize the final instrumentation construct. For cases in which pelvic fixation is required, the terminal end of the rod must often be bent aggressively; however, care must be taken to avoid angularities that might prevent rod passage between screw extensions. As with any multilevel construct, a softly contoured rod allows for smooth transitions. To ensure proper contouring, the rod may be laid directly on the patient's body or the screw extensions.

TECHNICAL CONSIDERATIONS
Spinal Pathology and Anatomic Challenges

Surgeons must be aware of any previous laminectomy performed on a spine to prevent introduction of the rod into the spinal canal. Moreover, one must consider the shingling effects of the posterior morphology of the thoracic and lumbar lamina. Because of this anatomy, a protective effect is created superiorly over the spinal canal and neural elements. Thus, surgeons should attempt to pass the rod from cranial to caudal. Additionally, when larger coronal and/or sagittal plane deformities are instrumented, surgeons should consider the risks of inadvertent rod placement into the chest or even the retroperitoneal space. If rod passage does not have a smooth transition, immediate fluoroscopic imaging should be considered to assist guiding the rod into the proper trajectory. If the rod enters the chest or abdominal cavity, further diagnostic workup should be undertaken to rule out injuries to vital structures.

Junctional Challenges

Performing minimally invasive fixation in the upper thoracic spine, just below the cervicothoracic junction, can be challenging. Adequate anteroposterior and lateral fluoroscopic imaging can be difficult because of body habitus and patient positioning. Because of the normal kyphosis in the upper thoracic spine associated with cervical lordosis and the cranium, placement of the patient's head in a skeletal pin holder headrest should be considered so that it may be placed in a somewhat flexed position. This placement allows the rod and rod holder to be manipulated through the upper screw extensions without navigating around the patient's head.

Difficulties typically arise when long constructs cross the thoracolumbar junction. The lordotic portion of the rod passes more easily across the thoracic kyphosis, but passage from the upper thoracic region toward the lumbosacral junction generally becomes more difficult as the kyphotic portion of the rod is passed across the thoracic apex. Typically, manipulation of the kyphotic portion of the rod into a more coronal plane or frank lordotic position facilitates the passage of the rod across the thoracic spine. Manipulating the rod with a Harrington rod holder assists the derotational maneuvers. Alternatively, implant manufacturers have developed rod inserters that allow in situ rotation of the rod, which can overcome these challenging issues (see Fig. 7-1).

CONCLUSION

Spine surgeons are now inserting multilevel, minimally invasive spinal constructs for conditions of the thoracolumbar spine such as tumors, trauma, infection, and adult and pediatric deformities. With the development of more advanced instrumentation, multilevel procedures have become easier to perform. Once spine surgeons have mastered performing one- and two-level rod passages, they will more easily be able to learn more-advanced, multilevel techniques.

SURGICAL PEARLS AND PITFALLS

- Before rod placement, screw entry points should be chosen carefully, and screw heights should be adjusted so that final rod insertion is straightforward.

- Some bend in the rod tip is helpful to guide the rod medially and laterally.

- Guiding the rod medially and laterally is accomplished best by rotating it about its long axis.

- Aggressive bends in the rod make passage difficult.

- It is generally easier to pass a rod through a construct from cranial to caudal.

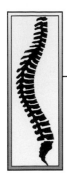

8

Potential Complications and Postoperative Care

Michael Y. Wang, Robert W. Irwin

Minimally invasive spinal instrumentation procedures are intended to reduce the pain and disability that patients experience during recovery compared with open procedures. Nevertheless, minimally invasive surgery (MIS) is a major procedure. Most patients need to be hospitalized for intravenous pain medications, observation, wound care, and nursing assistance until physical and occupational therapists confirm that the patient can be discharged. Although many of the protocols for avoiding complications and managing postoperative care used for open surgery also apply to MIS, some features of MIS are unique, and these differences are worth noting.

PREVENTING INFECTION

One of the major advantages of MIS of the spine is a lower rate of wound infection, which is attributed to numerous factors. First, the amount of soft tissue devascularization is reduced, thus preserving the body's wound-healing capacities. Second, the operative site has minimal dead space. This reduces the physical space available for infection or abscess formation, and it also promotes healthy muscle contact with the implants, minimizing the ability of bacteria to accumulate a glycocalyx or slime layer on the implants. Third, reduced intraoperative bleeding typically results in less seroma accumulation, which is another potential nidus for foreign organisms.

In a recent review of percutaneous thoracolumbar instrumentation conducted at nine collaborating institutions, overall infection rates were found to be lower than those of historical controls.[1] The review included 437 surgeries performed over a 3-year period that implanted a total of 2204 screws. Follow-up averaged 13.8 months. One superficial infection was identified, yielding an overall rate of 0.2% (Fig. 8-1).

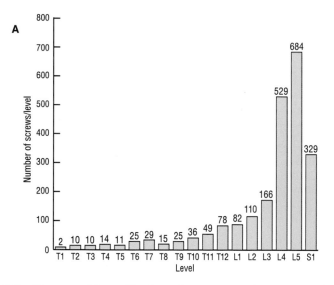

FIG. 8-1   Demographic profile of a multi-institutional case series of 437 patients treated with 2204 screws. The overall infection rate was 0.2%. **A,** Numbers and locations of inserted screws.

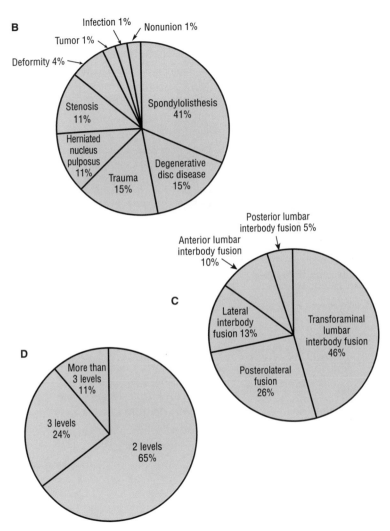

FIG. 8-1, cont'd B, Indications for surgery. C, Type of procedure. D, Number of levels fused.

MANAGING MUSCLE SPASM

Although muscle devitalization and destruction are reduced with a minimally invasive approach, leaving the muscles intact can have an unintended effect in some patients. Retraction with a tubular dilator, percutaneous screw placement, and subfascial rod passage cause soft tissue irritation that can be intensely painful. Younger male patients are particularly prone to this problem. The pain is self-limiting, but it can result in prolonged hospitalization or conflict with the patient's expectations of an MIS procedure.

Table 8-1
Common Medications for Reducing Postoperative Muscle Spasm

Medication (Trade Name)	Mechanism of Action
Cyclobenzaprine (Flexeril)	Unclear, but structurally similar to tricyclic antidepressants; activates the locus caeruleus in the brainstem, leading to an increased release of norepinephrine in the ventral horn of the spinal cord and the subsequent inhibitory action of norepinephrine on alpha motor neurons
Diazepam (Valium)	Benzodiazepine interacting with the GABA-A receptor

*Doses may vary, depending on the practitioner, patient variables, and institutional protocols.
GABA, Gamma-aminobutyric acid.

If left untreated, spasms may last from a few days to several weeks. The problem is best managed medically with nonnarcotic agents. A variety of muscle relaxants (rather than narcotic agents) can be useful, as shown in Table 8-1. For patients with persistent pain, bracing and physical treatments such as heat or ice, massage, and ultrasound can be helpful. Extreme cases may benefit from an injection of *botulinum* toxin, but, because of the cost of this product and the self-limiting nature of the disorder, this is rarely necessary.

Dose*	Adverse Effects
5-10 mg PO tid (start with a low dose in elderly patients)	Drowsiness, dry mouth, and dizziness
1-10 mg IV/IM/PO/PR q6-8h	Sedation, respiratory depression, addiction, physical dependence, and withdrawal; benzodiazepines require special precautions with alcohol- or drug-dependent individuals and elderly patients

Continued

Table 8-1—cont'd
Common Medications for Reducing Postoperative Muscle Spasm

Medication (Trade Name)	Mechanism of Action
Lorazepam (Ativan)	Lorazepam is a benzodiazepine that interacts with the GABA-A receptor (shorter acting)
Baclofen (Lioresal)	GABA (inhibitory) neurotransmitter analog modulating the GABA-B receptor, similar to the drug GHB
Carisoprodol (Soma)	Centrally acting skeletal muscle relaxant
Methocarbamol (Robaxin)	Central muscle relaxant
Metaxalone (Skelaxin)	Unknown, but it may be general central nervous system depression

*Doses may vary, depending on the practitioner, patient variables, and institutional protocols.
GHB, Gamma-hydroxybutyrate.

Dose*	Adverse Effects
0.5-2 mg IV/IM/PO q8h	Sedation, respiratory depression, addiction, physical dependence, and withdrawal; benzodiazepines require special precaution if used in alcohol- or drug-dependent individuals and elderly patients
5-20 mg PO tid (increase slowly)	Muscle fatigue, weakness, sedation, constipation, headache, increased salivation, withdrawal seizures, urinary retention; abrupt discontinuation can be associated with a withdrawal syndrome resembling benzodiazepine or alcohol withdrawal (more likely if baclofen is used for long periods of time); the dose should be tapered off slowly when discontinuing baclofen therapy; withdrawal symptoms may include hallucinations, confusion, agitation, delirium, memory impairments, psychosis, tachycardia, seizures, autonomic dysfunction, hyperpyrexia, extreme muscle rigidity, and rebound spasticity
250-350 mg PO tid	Drowsiness, dizziness, headache, addiction potential, and lowers seizure threshold
1000-1500 mg PO tid to qid	Stomach upset, nausea, flushing, constipation, headache, blurred vision, light-headedness, dizziness, drowsiness, and lowers seizure threshold
800 mg PO tid to qid	Dizziness, drowsiness, headache, irritability, nausea, nervousness, upset stomach, and vomiting

WOUND CARE, HEALING, AND COSMESIS

Because one of the potential benefits of MIS is a smaller incision, many patients expect improved cosmesis with these procedures compared with traditional open surgeries (Fig. 8-2). Reduced tissue and epidermal trauma inherently results in better scarring, and this can be particularly important in darker-skinned individuals or those prone to keloid formation.

Wound management begins in the operating room during surgical planning. Injecting local anesthetic into the dermis expands the skin before it is incised and creates a peau d'orange appearance (injection of the deeper layers does not have this effect). This effect results in a 25% to 30% expansion of the skin, which resolves after the surgery has been completed, thus resulting in a similar net decrease in the incision length and scar. Because clean incisions tend to heal better, we use a No. 10 scalpel blade and minimize

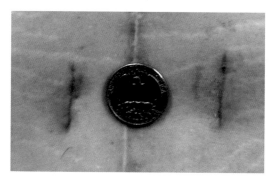

FIG. 8-2   A patient with previous midline exposure for laminectomy. The size of the incision is compared against two laterally placed incisions for a minimally invasive approach for instrumented fusion.

monopolar cautery directly on the skin. We also prefer to make the incision large enough to cause minimal epidermal stretching with the tubular dilator retractors. A small incision that is stretched during tubular retractor placement will undergo retractor burn, with the surrounding tissues appearing dusky—and even necrotic—by the end of a long case. This ultimately results in poor cosmesis, even if the incision length is shorter.

Closure is best performed with a small-diameter resorbable monofilament suture, such as 3-0 or 4-0 undyed Monocryl, buried in the dermis using a continuous subcuticular technique (Fig. 8-3). Knotted ends can be buried. However, for cases in which cosmesis is of high importance or keloid formation is likely, the ends can be left outside the body and removed 4 to 7 days after surgery, minimizing the presence of foreign body materials close to the skin surface.

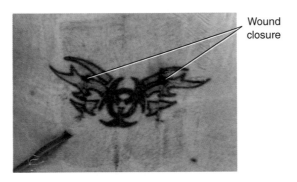

Wound closure

FIG. 8-3   Careful closure with a subcuticular resorbable suture and cyano-acrylate skin glue provide an excellent cosmetic result.

Postoperatively, the wound is kept dry and covered. Cyano-acrylate glue, such as Dermabond, is used on the skin in most patients, serving as a semiocclusive barrier that also reduces stress on the skin. This polymer barrier is left undisturbed until it falls off 2 to 4 weeks after surgery. At that point, patients are encouraged to apply creams that will help reduce superficial scar formation and improve cosmesis.

MOBILIZATION AND BRACING

Postoperatively, patients should be mobilized rapidly to minimize the risk of venous thromboembolism, atelectasis, pneumonia, and skin breakdown. In cases with long-segment fixation, osteopenia, or compromised fixation, an external orthosis should be used. Physical and occupational therapy can be beneficial, particularly for patients who are deconditioned preoperatively. Therapy can also help patients learn appropriate activities to minimize the risk of construct failure or nonunion.

PROMOTING FUSION

Intraoperatively, adequate preparation of the graft recipient site, whether interbody or posterolateral, followed by proper use of graft materials, is vital for ensuring the highest chance for a successful arthrodesis. Postoperatively, several measures can be used for maximizing the chances for fusion. Systemic assessment of the patient's nutritional status is vital for both soft tissue and bony healing. Protein and vitamins should be supplemented through a balanced diet or protein shakes. Protein is necessary for soft tissue regrowth, and high doses of vitamin C allow proper collagen formation. Bone formation is promoted with adequate doses of calcium and vitamin D, which is frequently deficient in spine fusion patients. Patients should be cautioned about the risks cigarette smoking poses to bone regrowth and fusion (see Chapter 9).

Bisphosphonates, which are ordinarily very helpful for treating osteoporosis, should be avoided because of their adverse effect on bone regrowth and remodeling.

Electrical bone stimulation can promote fusion in specific cases. They create a local magnetic field that promotes bone growth. Osteocytes and osteoblasts have a dipole orientation and respond to magnetic fields with increased growth and extracellular matrix deposition. Devices for this can be implanted but are more commonly applied externally. External devices can be worn as an orthosis or applied with adhesive leads to the skin (Fig. 8-4).

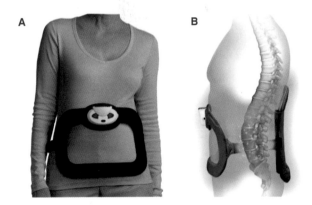

FIG. 8-4   **A,** An external bone stimulator device is implemented using an external orthosis. **B,** The area affected electromagnetically by the bone stimulator device is shown. (Images courtesy of Orthofix Holdings, Inc.)

Controlling Osteobiologics

Bone fusion adjuvants have become popular over the past decade. These substances, designed to promote fusion without the use of autologous iliac crest bone, have been fundamental in promoting successful minimally invasive spine fusions. Cadaveric allograft, demineralized bone matrices and putties, platelet-rich plasma concentrates, bone marrow aspirates, hydroxyapatite, ceramics, and silicate products have all become commercially available for the purpose of promoting fusion.

Recombinant bone morphogenetic proteins (BMPs) have been particularly useful for enhancing the likelihood of successful arthrodesis. BMP-2 (InFuse, Medtronic Sofamor Danek, Memphis, TN) and BMP-7 (OP-1, Stryker Biologics, Hopkinton, MA) have recently become commercially available. Although experience with rhBMP-7 has been limited, off-label use of rhBMP-2 is more common. The use of rhBMP-2 has led to strikingly higher fusion rates, but new complications are possible. Osteolysis, interbody settling, and seroma formation have been reported. However, there is minimal dead space with MIS, and wound drains are used infrequently. Thus sterile seromas can form under high pressure, causing an intense radiculitis that begins 4 to 14 days after surgery and lasts for days to weeks (Fig. 8-5). Drainage or needle aspiration, in conjunction with antiinflammatory medications, appears to be the best method for managing this sequela.

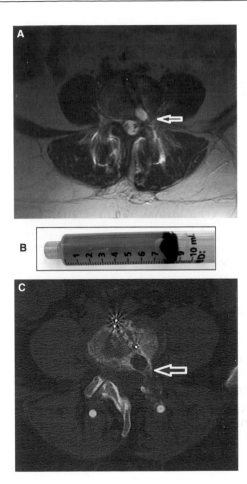

FIG. 8-5 A 56-year-old woman underwent a single-level minimally invasive TLIF. She did well postoperatively, but developed new sciatic pain. **A,** An MRI scan showed a cyst *(arrow)* from which clear sterile fluid was aspirated. **B,** The volume of aspirate was greater than that indicated from the MRI and was under high pressure. The patient's symptoms recurred. **C,** A CT scan revealed a calcified cyst that, on reexploration, was discovered to be an eggshell-thin layer of bone impinging on the traversing nerve root *(arrow)*.

CONCLUSION

MIS can frequently simplify the postoperative course for spine patients. However, there are some new and unique differences associated with these new methods that are based on the specific technique, implants, and pharmacologic agents used. Surgeons applying MIS methods must adapt specific regimens to accommodate these new procedures.

Reference

1. Hoh DJ, Anderson DG, Massey C, Tannoury T, Macko J, Wang MY. Multi-center study of the safety and durability of cannulated pedicle screws placed for percutaneous spinal stabilization. Presented at the Congress of Neurological Surgeons, Orlando, FL, Sept 2008.

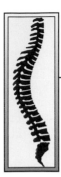

9

Achieving a Successful Fusion

Andrew C. Roeser, Praveen V. Mummaneni

To achieve a successful fusion, spine surgeons must pay close attention not only to placing instrumentation but also to bone graft placement. The fusion portion of a procedure often occurs at the end of a long surgery of placing instrumentation and can seem like an afterthought. However, bone graft placement is just as critical as appropriate hardware placement for achieving good long-term results.

The options for bone graft placement in MIS may be restricted by the limited exposure. In the lumbar spine, the three areas commonly incorporated into the fusion are the interbody space, the facet joint, and the intertransverse process region.

GRAFT MATERIALS AND AGENTS

There are three components of bone healing and fusion: osteogenesis, osteoinduction, and osteoconduction. Osteogenesis forms bone at a cellular (osteoblastic) level through the activity of osteoprogenitor stem cells. Osteoinduction enhances bone formation by recruiting and inducing undifferentiated tissue to differentiate into bone. Osteoconduction creates scaffolding to guide the growth of closely apposed, growing and healing bone.

Autografts are the benchmark strategy for attaining bone fusion. They provide the osteogenic, osteoinductive, and osteoconductive components required to achieve fusion. Allografts provide only an osteoconductive scaffolding. Demineralized bone matrixes (DBMs) are theoretically composed of osteoinductive agents, but they provide no support.

Interbody spacers and strut grafts provide immediate stability and structural integrity. They can be packed with other bone-forming materials (such as an autograft) to create fusion.

Synthetic bone substitutes, such as hydroxyapatite, work similarly to allografts in that they are primarily osteoinductive: they create a scaffold that supports cell attachment and bony ingrowth. Sometimes the grafts are soaked in bone marrow aspirate taken during the procedure to supplement the scaffolding activity.

Bioactive agents have been developed that take advantage of osteoinduction or osteogenesis. The most commonly used bioactive agent is recombinant human bone morphogenic protein (rhBMP-2). This protein works by osteoinduction—enhancing factors in the fusion pathway—and it is approved by the FDA for use in anterior lumbar fusion procedures. Other strategies involving stem cells and gene therapy are also being developed.

PREOPERATIVE PLANNING

A patient's physical examination, radiographic imaging, and medical history aid in determining systemic and local factors that may affect surgical fusion.

Patient Evaluation

A thorough history helps define systemic factors, such as diseases, medications, and social habits, that may hinder arthrodesis. For example, patients with severe osteopenia or osteoporosis are more likely to develop a pseudarthrosis. This condition may be idiopathic or related to a medical condition (such as Cushing's disease, parathyroid disease, or renal failure). Pseudarthrosis in these patients may be caused by a decreased number of osteogenic stem cells rather than absolute bone mass.[1] A bone density scan with a focus on the lumbar spine can help quantify the bone quality. These patients may benefit from perioperative anabolic medications such as teriparatide (Forteo) to help strengthen and build bone.[2]

Other important variables include cigarette smoking and medication use. Patients who smoke have a higher risk for pseudarthrosis than those who do not. Cigarette smoking retards osteogenesis and inhibits graft revascularization. Silcox et al[3] showed a direct relationship between systemic nicotine and spinal pseudarthrosis in a rat model. Smoking cessation before surgery and up to 6 months postoperatively is recommended.

Drugs taken during the perioperative period can also have a detrimental effect on spinal fusion. Chemotherapeutic agents and nonsteroidal antiinflammatory drugs (NSAIDs) both suppress the inflammatory response and may inhibit fusion. Corticosteroids have been shown to increase bone resorption and decrease new bone formation, both experimentally and clinically.[4-6] Ideally, anti-inflammatory drug use should be discontinued temporarily before fusion surgery, and resumption of such medications (especially aspirin) should be avoided until there is radiologic evidence of fusion.[7]

Radiographic Workup

Imaging studies are ordered according to the patient's symptoms and clinical diagnosis. In the lumbar spine, flexion-extension radiograph, MRI, CT, or CT myelogram studies are commonly performed. Radiographs and CT scans can provide an overall sense of a patient's bone quality and the anatomy of the fusion environment. Patients with radiographically poor bone quality should be considered for further study with a bone density scan. A collapsed and sclerotic disc space may make TLIF more difficult. The size (or absence) of transverse processes may affect posterolateral arthrodesis. Autofusion of spinal segments may also occur if there is degenerative spine disease, and this should be taken into consideration.

Patients with scoliosis should undergo a standing, 36-inch, scoliosis radiograph series. Extending the fusion to correct kyphoscoliosis and restore spinal balance in the sagittal plane is critical for achieving good long-term outcomes. Failure to take spinal balance into consideration can result in worsening of the deformity and adjacent segment disease.

Disc space height in the lower lumbar region (L4-5 and L5-S1) can also affect the chances of achieving successful fusion. Patients with large discs in this area retain a significant amount of motion, and posterolateral arthrodesis by itself is often insufficient for achieving fusion in these high-stress regions. Posterior interbody fusion (PLIF/TLIF) or ALIF procedures should be considered for

these patients. This is especially true in patients with spondylo-
lysis, because absence of the pars may hinder the creation of a robust posterolateral fusion mass.

Bone Graft

Planning for the type of bone graft to be used should be done before surgery. An allograft may be chosen for the interbody space,
but they do not work well in the posterolateral gutters. Bone graft
extenders may be used in ALIF procedures; however, we prefer
iliac autograft for most procedures. Make sure that appropriate
autograft harvesting tools are available before starting the procedure. Preparation helps streamline the process and avoids chang-
ing the operative plan or waiting.

SURGICAL TECHNIQUE

Adequate preparation of the graft recipient site and proper use of
graft materials are crucial for successful fusion.

Patient Positioning and Bone Graft Harvesting

Our preferred method for minimally invasive posterior lumbar fusion is TLIF. The patient is placed on a Wilson frame that is set in
the upmost position during the exposure and decompression portion of the procedure and then lowered to restore lumbar lordosis
before securing the spine with instrumentation. A skin incision is
made 2 to 3 fingerbreadths from the midline on the side where
the decompression/TLIF is to be performed, and it should be long
enough to insert the MIS retractor (typically 3 cm). In low lumbar
procedures, iliac crest bone autograft is harvested through the in-

cision before placing the retractor. This is done by dissecting epifascially and inferolaterally toward the crest (Fig. 9-1). The iliac crest is exposed with the Bovie electrocautery. Either a handheld retractor or the MIS retractor can be used to maintain the exposure. Bone is removed with a quarter-inch osteotome and large-cup curettes. Cancellous bone is harvested preferentially over cortical bone.

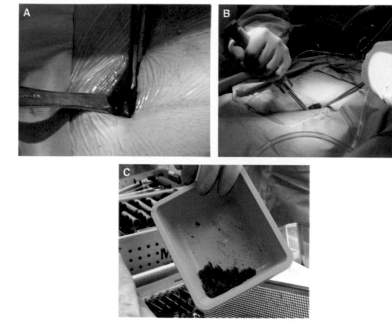

FIG. 9-1   **A,** A left paramedian incision is made for a minimally invasive TLIF procedure. Before inserting the muscle dilators, iliac crest bone graft is harvested. **B,** With a handheld retractor in place, an osteotome is used to begin graft removal. **C,** A sufficient amount of bone graft can easily be removed through this approach.

Facetectomy

The fascia is then opened, and the paraspinal muscles are serially dilated. The expandable tubular retractor is redirected and centered over the facet joint at the intended fusion level. After the joint is exposed, soft tissue is removed from its surface. A facetectomy is then performed using an osteotome or drill. First, the overlying superior facet is removed, followed by the inferior facet. Care should be taken not to violate the pedicles when removing the facet, and fluoroscopy may be helpful to identify the pedicle positions. It is often helpful to place the superior pedicle screw and tap the inferior pedicle before performing the facetectomy to help visualize where the pedicles are in relation to the facet joint. We do not place the inferior screw until later in the procedure to avoid obscuring visualization of the facet through the small tubular retractor. The bone harvested from the facetectomy is saved and prepared for use in the fusion mass.

Discectomy and Endplate Preparation

After facet removal, an aggressive discectomy is performed at the intended TLIF level. After the discectomy is performed, it is important to take sufficient time for endplate preparation. The endplate cartilage and the disc are removed by using progressively larger endplate shavers. Additionally, ringed curettes and endplate rasps are used to decorticate the interbody surfaces.

Cage and Bone Graft Placement

Trial cage spacers are placed to find the appropriate cage size, which is then packed with iliac crest autograft. Before placing the cage, the interbody space is partially filled with iliac crest autograft, which is pushed contralaterally and anteriorly within the disc space; then the cage packed with the autograft is placed. The area is irrigated with antibiotic solution before the bone graft is placed. Any remaining bone can be placed along the transverse processes after they have been decorticated.

In some cases, a posterolateral fusion may be performed on the side contralateral to the TLIF or PLIF. Alternatively, following an ALIF procedure, a posterolateral fusion may be performed dorsally. If this is done, the surgeon may place bone into the facet joints through a small port placed over the facet joint. The joint also may be decorticated with a drill placed through this small tubular retractor (Fig. 9-2). Bone graft may be placed into the decorticated facet joint, and the retractor is removed. Percutaneous pedicle screw fixation may then be performed (see Chapters 3 and 4).

Some surgeons prefer to use an expandable tubular retractor when performing a posterolateral fusion (Fig. 9-3). The expandable tubular retractor provides access not only to the facet joint but also to the medial transverse process area. The drill can be used to decorticate the facet joint as well as the transverse processes. Bone graft may then be placed into the facet joint and/or onto the transverse processes using a small bone funnel (Fig. 9-4). Subsequently, pedicle screw fixation may be performed through an expandable tubular retractor as well (see Chapter 5).

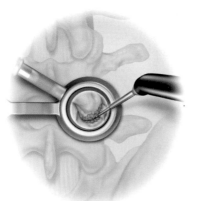

FIG. 9-2   A nonexpandable port retractor can be used to access and decorticate the facet joint with a drill. (Image © DePuy Spine, Inc. 2010. All rights reserved. Used with permission.)

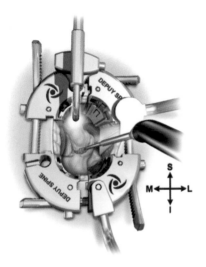

FIG. 9-3 An expandable tubular retractor is used to access the facet joint and the medial transverse processes. The facet joint is decorticated with a drill, and a channel can be cut into the facet joint to create space to place bone graft. Using an expandable tubular retractor, it is also possible to access and decorticate the transverse processes and to place pedicle screws (not shown). (Image © DePuy Spine, Inc. 2010. All rights reserved. Used with permission.)

FIG. 9-4 A bone funnel may be used to place bone graft into the channel created in the decorticated facet joint. (Image © DePuy Spine, Inc. 2010. All rights reserved. Used with permission.)

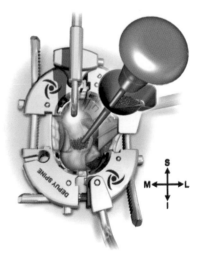

COMPLICATIONS

Complications of bone grafting include iliac harvest site infection and donor site pain. We typically pulse lavage the iliac crest area where the bone graft was harvested and leave a subfascial drain in place for 1 to 2 days. Failure of a graft to form a fusion (pseudarthrosis) is a delayed complication. We typically follow all of our patients for 2 years after surgery. Not all who develop radiographic pseudarthrosis have symptoms related to the bony nonunion. However, pseudarthrosis can lead to screw loosening and migration or instrumentation breakage.

CONCLUSION

Surgeons must ensure that adequate bone grafting is done in MIS cases. The hardware will loosen over time if the patient does not achieve a solid fusion.

SURGICAL PEARLS AND PITFALLS

- Take time to prepare the fusion bed properly.
- Place adequate bone graft to achieve fusion.

BAILOUTS/ALTERNATIVE STRATEGIES

- If there is inadequate autograft bone, consider using bone graft extenders (such as allograft).

References

1. Jergensen HE, Chua J, Kao RT, et al. Age effects on bone induction by demineralized bone powder. Clin Orthop Relat Res 268:253-259, 1991.
2. O'Loughlin PF, Cunningham ME, Bukata SV, et al. Parathyroid hormone (1-34) augments spinal fusion, fusion mass volume, and fusion mass quality in a rabbit spinal fusion model. Spine 34:121-130, 2009.
3. Silcox DH III, Daftari T, Boden SD, et al. The effect of nicotine on spinal fusion. Spine 20:1549-1553, 1995.
4. Cruess RL, Sakai T. Effect of cortisone upon synthesis rates of some components of rat bone matrix. Clin Orthop Relat Res 86:253-259, 1972.
5. Hahn TJ. Corticosteroid-induced osteopenia. Arch Intern Med 138: 882-885, 1978.
6. Jowsey J, Riggs BL. Bone formation in hypercortisonism. Acta Endocrinol (Copenh) 63:21-28, 1970.
7. Glassman SD, Rose SM, Dimar JR, et al. The effect of postoperative nonsteroidal anti-inflammatory drug administration on spinal fusion. Spine 23:834-838, 1998.

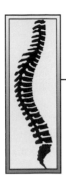

10

Pedicle Cannulation in Challenging Cases

Michael Y. Wang

Since its original description by Roy-Camille and Saillant,[1] transpedicular screw fixation remains the most widely accepted method for rigid segmental instrumentation of the thoracolumbar spine. The three-dimensional rigidity afforded by pedicle screw–rod constructs allows versatile and effective stabilization for treating degenerative, traumatic, infectious, and neoplastic disorders of the spine.

Percutaneous techniques for screw placement have been available and widely used in Europe for more than a decade to treat traumatic thoracolumbar injuries with temporary fracture fixation.[2,3] However, truly percutaneous subfascial screw-rod systems have only recently become available.[4-6] Although these systems have already evolved into their second and third design iterations, they account for less than 10% of the transpedicular screws used in the United States. Frequently, surgeons prefer to use an open procedure, because pedicle screw placement can be more straight-forward with this method.

However, percutaneous screw insertion under image guidance or fluoroscopy can be as accurate as open methods, provided specific principles and techniques are followed. Fundamental elements of intraoperative imaging and the various accepted cannulation techniques for straightforward cases are described elsewhere in this handbook. However, certain situations require particular adaptations of the technique for pedicle tract preparation to ensure proper screw placement. These are discussed here.

PREOPERATIVE PLANNING

Assessment and Evaluation

Understanding not only the general thoracolumbar spine anatomy, but also the bony features unique to each patient, is necessary in difficult cases. Preoperative CT scans are useful for outlining the bony anatomy of the lateral mass, and they can guide the surgeon to the projections of the pedicle, spinal canal, and overlying facet joints. The dorsal topography of the ideal screw entry points for each level and side should be noted, with particular attention to any bony prominences, asymmetries, and sclerosis. In addition, variations in vertebral body morphology determine the maximum screw length with any given transpedicular trajectory or angulation (Fig. 10-1).

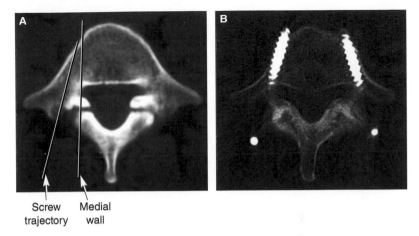

Screw   Medial
trajectory   wall

FIG. 10-1 **A,** A triangular lumbar vertebral body, requiring careful attention to the pedicle screw trajectory to avoid a pedicle breach or a prominent anterior screw, serves as an example of how preoperative CT scanning can be helpful. In this case, a more lateral starting point and 40-degree medialization are necessary to align the screw trajectory with the pedicle. A more medial starting point risks a pedicle breach near the nerve root. A lateral starting point with inadequate medialization (as shown here) requires shorter screws to prevent entry into the soft tissue spaces ventral to the vertebral body. Reduced tactile feedback during percutaneous techniques increases the risk of this problem. **B,** Lack of tactile feedback also introduces the possibility of inadvertent K-wire or screw entry into the retroperitoneum or peritoneal space.

Patient Positioning

It is critical for the patient to be positioned properly so that the Jamshidi needle can be placed safely and efficiently. We prefer to position the patient on a Jackson table, because other nonradiolucent tables can obstruct radiographic visualization (Fig. 10-2). In addition, the base of the typical operating room table can prevent proper AP or sagittal imaging, particularly when biplanar imaging is desired and a substantial amount of equipment footprint is involved.

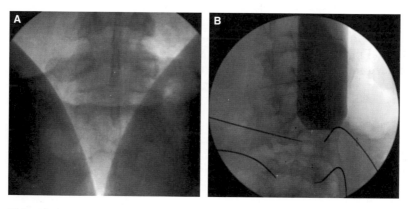

FIG. 10-2   **A,** A standard table with bolsters to enhance lordotic positioning obstructs the fluoroscopic view of the S1 pedicles. **B,** If the patient is short, a Mayfield head holder extension can obstruct the view of the upper thoracolumbar spine.

SMALL PEDICLE DIAMETERS

The anatomy of the thoracolumbar pedicles can pose specific challenges to screw placement. If preoperative CT scans reveal a small pedicle diameter, then the surgeon will have to pursue strategies for screw positioning near the nerve roots. This is most common at the L1 and L2 levels where the medial-lateral dimensions of the pedicles can be too small to accept a standard pedicle screw. In open surgery, exposure of the screw insertion point allows the surgeon to use anatomic landmarks to gauge the appropriate starting site. In addition, a laminectomy permits direct inspection of the medial pedicle wall and neighboring nerve root to ensure that there is no neural impingement.

For percutaneous screw placement, targeting the screw entry point on the medial transverse process results in an intentional lateral pedicle breach. A pedicle screw can thus be successfully placed into pedicles as small as 4 mm in diameter. This rarely results in nerve root irritation, given the distant location of the neural elements, and is preferable to a medial breach. However, a breach may already have occurred during Jamshidi needle placement. In this situation, the needle must be directed to re-enter the vertebral body. This is akin to the in-out-in method for thoracic pedicle screws, except that there is no rib head to cover the lateral breach. Attention must be given to ensure that the needle does not skive around the lateral wall of the vertebral body, or the screw will lie within the psoas muscle. A beveled needle tip may be helpful to redirect the tract into the vertebral body. Rotating the needle aligns the bevel, guiding the needle in a preferential direction.

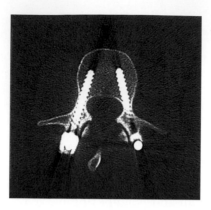

FIG. 10-3 This axial CT image shows placement of 6 mm pedicle screws into pedicles of exactly that diameter through a process of slow serial tap dilation. Notice that the pedicles are not sclerotic or otherwise prone to fracture.

For slightly larger pedicles, K-wire placement can be followed by serial bone dilation using sequentially larger taps. The ability of the pedicles to expand to a limited degree may allow the placement of screws equal to the diameter of the pedicles (Fig. 10-3). This technique should be avoided in patients with brittle or sclerotic bone, because there will be a tendency for a blowout fracture of the pedicle.

CANNULATION ADJACENT TO A TLIF

If a minimally invasive TLIF is being performed with pedicle cannulation, then several methods are available to ensure proper screw placement. Insertion of the screws under direct vision through a tubular dilator retractor (a mini-open approach; see Chapter 5) is similar to open surgery and can be a preferred technique for surgeons who desire tactile feedback and want to minimize intraoperative fluoroscopy.

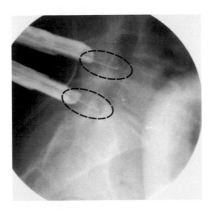

FIG. 10-4   Direct visualization of the pedicle after decompression through an expandable tubular retractor allows drilling the entry position for the pedicle screws, which in turn allows placement of flexible K-wires (*dashed circles*) into the pilot holes, followed by retractor removal. A Jamshidi needle is then placed over each K-wire and directed down the shaft of the pedicle using AP and lateral fluoroscopy. This eliminates difficulties obtaining a starting position on a sclerotic or overgrown facet joint, but also allows final trajectory determination using fluoroscopic guidance.

If Jamshidi cannulation is desired, then the laminotomy created for decompression and interbody cage placement can result in exiting nerve injury, because the defect allows easy, inadvertent instrument placement where bone has been removed. In addition, the discectomy and fusion site is just rostral to the lower pedicle, and drilling for lower exposure can lead to a steep slope off the pedicle projection, which tends to guide the needle into the disc space. One strategy for avoiding this problem involves drilling the needle entry points under direct vision through a tubular retractor (Fig. 10-4). This allows placement of a K-wire superficially through the retractor, followed by retractor removal. The Jamshidi needle can then be placed under fluoroscopy for ideal screw placement, with the starting point already predetermined and well situated.

LARGE OVERLYING FACET JOINTS

One of the most common obstacles to pedicle cannulation is a large overlying facet joint with sclerotic bone. This is a common situation, because segments to be fused are frequently affected by degenerative osteoarthritis (Fig. 10-5).

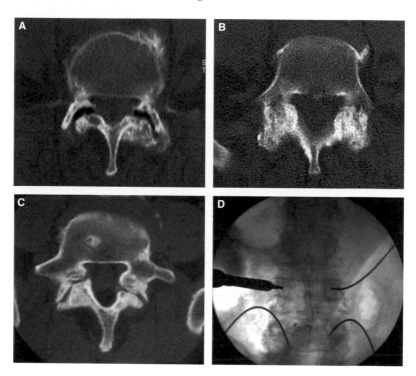

FIG. 10-5 Hypertrophic, sclerotic facets can be difficult starting points for percutaneous screws, whether caused by **A,** degeneration, or **B,** low-grade spondylolisthesis, or **C,** high-grade spondylolisthesis. **D,** A burr may be placed at the ideal starting surface through a small skin incision. The burr penetrates the sclerotic cortical bone and provides a depression on which to place the Jamshidi needles.

Degenerative spondylolistheses also results in associated hypertrophied facet joints. In this situation, the ideal starting point may be at the apex of a bony prominence, where anchoring with a Jamshidi needle is difficult and can lead to repeated failed attempts, because the needle tends to slip laterally. In open surgery, placing a burr on the ideal starting point provides an easy remedy. For percutaneous surgery, the same technique can be used by inserting the burr through the incision to create an entry point at a bony apex or through sclerotic bone under fluoroscopic guidance. Once this stable docking point has been created for needle entry, the rest of the cannulation can be performed more easily. Care must be taken to make a bony hole large enough that the surgeon can find it easily using a Jamshidi needle, without direct visualization.

CANNULATION WHEN OPTIMAL IMAGING CANNOT BE OBTAINED EASILY

Because percutaneous surgery is so dependent on intraoperative imaging to compensate for the lack of direct visualization, it is necessary to obtain high-quality radiographs of the bony anatomy. In cases involving spondylolisthesis or a Gill body, the pedicle outline can be difficult to visualize (Fig. 10-6). The medial pedicle wall may need to be inferred from the adjacent levels above and below. Alternatively, an en face, or oblique owl's eye, projection may give the surgeon a better appreciation of the bony anatomy (see Chapter 4). In these cases, the pedicle is also often small or sclerotic.

Similarly, appreciating the first sacral pedicle can also be difficult. This pedicle has a different three-dimensional configuration, and the projection on an AP view is typically that of a reverse or upside-down J, as shown in Fig. 10-7. The depth of this vertebral body along the cannulation trajectory can also be difficult to determine. We prefer to use tactile feedback to localize the anterior vertebral cortex at the site where the harder cortical bone increases resistance to Jamshidi needle and tap entry.

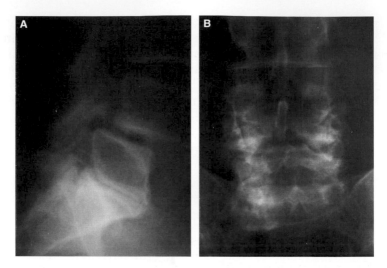

FIG. 10-6   A, Lateral and, B, AP radiographs showing the difficulty of imaging a pedicle near a spondylolisthesis.

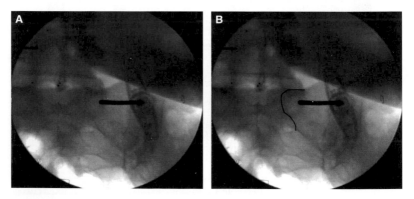

FIG. 10-7   Direct AP projection of the sacrum. A, The Jamshidi needle is in place. B, The medial outline of the S1 pedicle is highlighted.

OSTEOPOROTIC BONE

Although cannulating weak bone is often easier initially, control of the instruments is more difficult because of the lower resistance of osteoporotic bone. Inadvertent K-wire violation of the anterior vertebral body can injure the retroperitoneal structures. This is uncommon, but it can cause significant hemorrhage if the arterial or venous structures are damaged. More commonly, pedicle wall fractures and endplate violations are prone to occur (Fig. 10-8). Pedicle violations occur most often through the superior wall, particularly if this area has been weakened during the decompression, or if a TLIF cage was placed with the assistance of a box chisel.

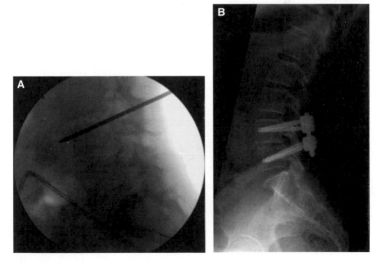

FIG. 10-8 **A,** Osteoporotic bone can present a challenge for needle control. In this case, overly aggressive malleting resulted in a superior pedicle breach, as well as needle entry past the anterior cortex and into the retroperitoneum. **B,** Endplate violations are also prone to occur, with cage migration into the inferior vertebral body.

Care must also be taken in patients with osteoporosis during reduction maneuvers or when trying to mate a screw saddle to a rod. Special attention must be given to placing screws with polyaxial heads in good alignment so that rod mating can be accomplished with minimal force. To correct a deformity or spondylolisthesis, the correction maneuvers should be performed in a manner that distributes the load over as many fixation points as possible. For example, spondylolistheses should be reduced slowly and with simultaneous bilateral forces.

CANNULATION FOLLOWING A PREVIOUSLY FAILED ATTEMPT

One of the most frustrating situations in percutaneous surgery involves recannulation of a pedicle after a suboptimal initial tract has already been created. If the entry point is suboptimal, then redrilling the shallow portion of the pilot hole with a burr is an option (see Fig. 10-5, *D*). If the entry point is acceptable but the trajectory is not optimal, a beveled Jamshidi needle allows the tract to be redirected by several degrees.

If more correction is desired, a cannulated pedicle probe (Fig. 10-9) can be a powerful means for redirecting the screw trajectory. This instrument essentially uses an open technique through a small skin incision to re-create a tract, allows greater forces to be

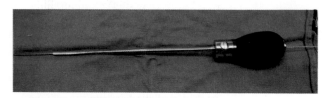

FIG. 10-9   A cannulated pedicle probe allows direct, tactile pedicle cannulation, followed by K-wire placement, permitting percutaneous pedicle screws to be used.

applied in all planes, and gives tactile feedback to the surgeon. The central hole in the instrument allows placement of a K-wire after successful cannulation. Screw placement is then performed in a typical fashion.

TREATING OBESE PATIENTS

Minimally invasive techniques have been promoted as potentially more advantageous for obese patients (Fig. 10-10). This may be true from a patient's perspective, but obese patients pose a greater challenge to the surgeon, in part because of the increased distance to the target, but also because of the reduced image quality created by the increased mass of surrounding soft tissues. One way to circumvent the distance problem is to make a larger skin incision (6 to 8 cm) and open the fatty tissues. The level of the fascia then becomes like the skin surface, allowing the tubular port to be sunk deeper into the body, or allowing the use of fixed tubes that do not have a larger outer frame. This method effectively reduces the distance to the target (facet joint or lamina) by 2 to 5 cm.

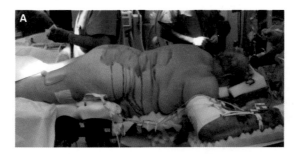

FIG. 10-10 A, The body habitus of this patient (who had a BMI of 42) made imaging problematic, and, although positioned on a Jackson table, the spine was axially rotated. This was compensated for by rotating the bed in the opposite direction. *Continued*

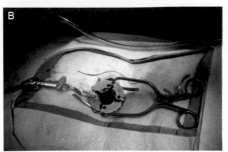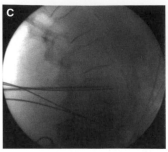

FIG. 10-10, cont'd   B, Making a large skin/fat incision allows the retractor to be placed within the fat, reducing the length of the tube that is needed. C, Intraoperative fluoroscopic view of K-wires crossing within the patient's dorsal musculature. This can result in snagging adjacent screw extensions or a K-wire.

A secondary issue with increased depth to the target is the need to make finer angular adjustments in needle positioning. As the depth increases beyond 12 cm, a small change in needle angulation results in a significant translation in location on the surface of the spine.

In addition, because of the lumbar lordosis in large patients, the K-wires, which typically cross outside the body, may cross within the patient's body. If this occurs, care must be exercised to keep track of which wire leads to which level, and to avoid snagging or entrapping the screws and their extensions when inserting them, because the wires may cross within the dorsal spinal musculature. With polyaxial screw extensions, which can pivot, the bulk of the metallic screw extensions can become entrapped.

SPINAL DEFORMITY AND CANNULATION

Minimally invasive techniques are of the most benefit for treating adult spinal deformities. Because of the severe medical comorbidities frequently seen in this patient population, surgery with a lower complication rate represents a significant treatment advance. Although still in its infancy, the correction of lower-grade degenerative curves and listhesis has become possible.[7]

These procedures are typically performed in two stages, with an initial lateral approach for discectomy, release, and interbody cage placement for fusion (Fig. 10-11), and a second stage for percutaneous screw placement and additional reduction maneuvers through rod derotation and compression/distraction between screw heads. The instrumentation for these procedures is still in its early stages, but it will probably undergo significant advances in the coming years.

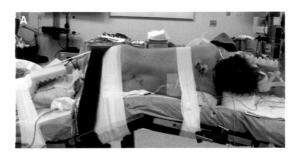

FIG. 10-11   Minimally invasive surgery for adult degenerative scoliosis. A, The first stage of surgery is performed with the patient in the lateral position, with access from the convex side.   *Continued*

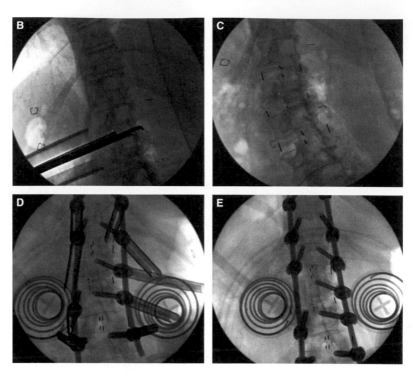

FIG. 10-11, cont'd B, Intervertebral release, distraction, and opening of the contralateral (concave) anulus. C, Cage placement. D, Percutaneous screw placement. E, Rod derotation and final deformity correction.

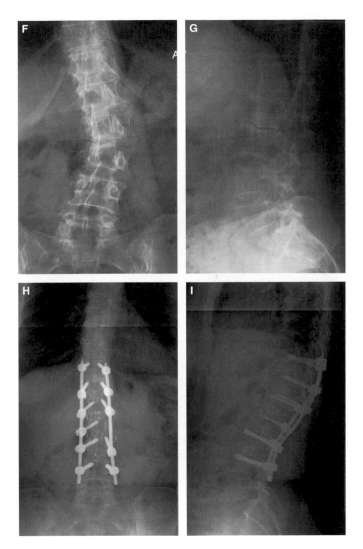

FIG. 10-11, cont'd   F and G, Preoperative images. H and I, Postoperative radiographs demonstrating correction of coronal and sagittal alignment.

CONCLUSION

The placement of percutaneous pedicle screws and rods can be achieved with a high degree of safety. The establishment of an efficient workflow is essential to shorten operative times, minimize surgeon fatigue, reduce radiation exposure, and maximize the potential for successful construct placement. The use of particular adaptive techniques to overcome common problems makes percutaneous instrumentation accessible to surgeons familiar with standard open stabilization procedures.

References
1. Roy-Camille R, Saillant G. Vertebral osteosynthesis using metal plates. Its different uses. Chirurgie 105:579-603, 1979.
2. Wiesner L, Kothe R, Ruther W. Anatomic evaluation of two different techniques for the percutaneous insertion of pedicle screws in the lumbar spine. Spine 24:1599-1603, 1999.
3. Wiesner L, Kothe R, Schulitz KP, et al. Clinical evaluation and computed tomography scan analysis after percutaneous insertion of pedicle screws in the lumbar spine. Spine 25:615-621, 2000.
4. Foley KT, Gupta SK. Percutaneous pedicle screw fixation in the lumbar spine: preliminary clinical results. J Neurosurg 97(1 Suppl):S7-S12, 2002.
5. Khoo LT, Palmer S, Laich DT, et al. Minimally invasive percutaneous posterior lumbar interbody fusion. Neurosurgery 51(5 Suppl):S166-S171, 2002.
6. Wang MY, Kim KA, Hoh DJ. Minimally invasive spinal surgery. Contemp Neurosurg 27:1-4, 2005.
7. Wang MY, Anderson DG, Poelstra KA, et al. Minimally invasive posterior fixation. Neurosurg 63:197-203, 2008.

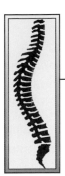

11

Pushing the Limits of Percutaneous Spine Fixation

Michael Y. Wang

During the past decade, a large number of new techniques and technologies for minimally invasive spine instrumentation and fusion have appeared. Although minimally invasive TLIF and lateral approaches, as well as percutaneous transpedicular screws, remain the cornerstone of minimally invasive thoracolumbar surgery, there are additional methods, as well as bailout strategies, for addressing special situations. This chapter addresses some, but not all, of these methods, with the understanding that this is a continually evolving field and that technology improvements occur regularly.

VERTEBRAL BODY AUGMENTATION

The use of polymethylmethacrylate (PMMA) cement to treat bony defects and fill bone-implant gaps has been a common orthopedic and neurosurgical practice for many decades.[1] The biologic safety of cement has been well validated, but its use in the spinal column is relatively new. Vertebroplasty was initially developed in France to treat bone neoplasms, but more recently it has become popular in the United States as a treatment for osteoporotic compression fractures. Kyphoplasty (inflating a balloon in the vertebral body to potentially restore anterior column height and create a cavity for cement injection) has also become popular (Fig. 11-1). Although controversial, most surgeons and the peer-reviewed literature indicate that vertebroplasty and kyphoplasty result in similar clinical outcomes.

The surgical procedure involves a transpedicular or parapedicular cannulation of the vertebral body with a Jamshidi needle. This is followed by cavity creation (with kyphoplasty) and PMMA cement injection. Great care must be taken to track the cement on AP and lateral fluoroscopic images to control and prevent any potential PMMA extravasation. Extrusion posteriorly into the spinal canal can be particularly dangerous, and care must be exercised in patients who have a burst fracture or break in the posterior vertebral wall (Fig. 11-2). Cement migration into the large vertebral veins followed by pulmonary embolism has also been reported.

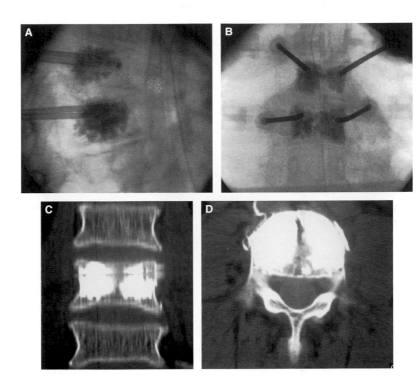

FIG. 11-1   **A** and **B**, Vertebroplasty with pedicle cannulation followed by PMMA cement injection under fluoroscopic guidance to avoid extravasation. **C** and **D**, Kyphoplasty includes balloon inflation to create a cavity in the vertebral body, resulting in dense cement filling of the space.

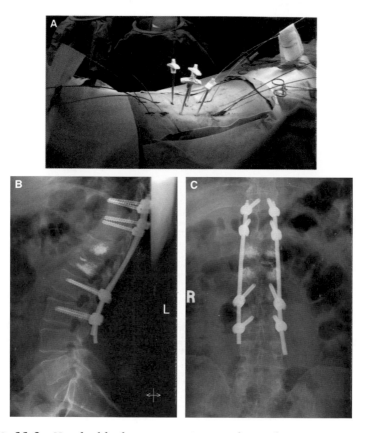

FIG. 11-2   Vertebral body augmentation together with percutaneous instrumentation in a patient suffering two-level burst fractures from trauma and osteoporosis. Great care must be exercised in such cases to prevent posterior cement extrusion into the spinal canal. A, Percutaneous cannulation of pedicles for K-wires (for pedicle screw tracts) and Jamshidi needles (for cement injection). B and C, Postoperative radiographs.

PEDICLE SCREW AUGMENTATION

For patients with severe osteopenia or osteoporosis, traditional cancellous pedicle screws may prove biomechanically inadequate. Options include avoiding implant placement altogether, prolonged postoperative bracing, use of larger-diameter screws, accomplishing bicortical screw purchase, and lengthening the construct.

The bone-screw interface can be enhanced with PMMA cement (Fig. 11-3). Although the PMMA-bone interface is at risk for breakdown, in select patients there may be no other options. The screw tracts may be injected after tapping and before screw placement.[2] For percutaneous screws, a vertebroplasty may be done, followed quickly by screw tapping and insertion before the cement polymerizes. Injection of the cement through fenestrated screws is an additional op-

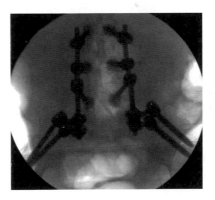

FIG. 11-3   PMMA augmentation to improve screw pullout strength in a case of a sacral insufficiency fracture from severe osteoporosis.

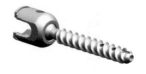

tion (Fig. 11-4). For cases using PMMA reinforcement, it is critical to finalize the screw insertion depth at each site before the cement hardens, because adjustments will be extremely difficult later.

ILIAC SCREW PLACEMENT

Percutaneous iliac screw insertion has recently been reported in the literature.[3] Large-diameter (7.0 to 10.0 mm) and long (65 to 120 mm) screws in the ilium allow stabilization of a construct well past the pivoting point of the lumbosacral junction. In this manner, iliac screw fixation is a powerful stabilizer in both the coronal and sagittal planes, and it is especially effective for long-segment constructs. In addition, percutaneous iliac screw insertion provides a useful salvage technique when S1 or S2 fixation is either inadequate or unavailable.

Percutaneous screw placement depends heavily on fluoroscopic imaging targeted at the ischial body. The *obturator outlet* view requires working closely with the radiologic technician to adjust the beam in two planes (Fig. 11-5). This view shows a direct projection of the ischial body, which is the intended location for the screw tip. By choosing a reasonable starting point and targeting the screw tip into the teardrop projection of the ischial body, the screw

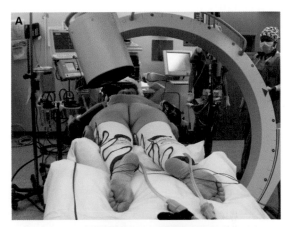

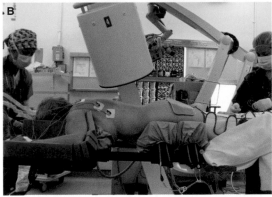

FIG. 11-5 Setting up the fluoroscope to obtain obturator outlet views. Notice the alignment in both the **A,** axial and **B,** sagittal planes to develop the proper teardrop view of the ischial body.

can be placed reliably using two-dimensional fluoroscopy (Fig. 11-6). One can also envision the target as the cancellous bone where the inner and outer tables of the medial and lateral aspects of the pelvis overlap. Because the pelvis is shaped like a bowl, the overlap point is in the inferior pelvis, and it is teardrop-shaped instead of being a quadrilateral.

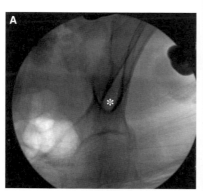
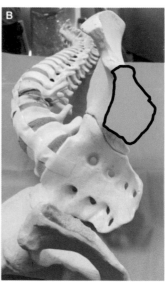

FIG. 11-6 A, Fluoroscopic view of the ischial body where the Jamshidi needle should be placed *(asterisk)*. B, Sawbones section showing the teardrop view of the ischial body *(outlined)*. This is the target for true percutaneous iliac screw placement.

The screw entry point can vary, but I generally prefer to enter at the recession below the posterior superior iliac spine (PSIS). Care must be taken to avoid entering the sacroiliac joint plane, which is possible if starting with a Jamshidi needle. The entry point can be prepared by osteotomizing a 1 by 1 cm square of bone to access the cancellous bone, and this can be accomplished through a 1.5 cm skin incision. This will allow proper recession of the screw head.

Screw placement then proceeds in the standard percutaneous fashion (Jamshidi needle placement, K-wire insertion, tapping, and palpation). Cannulated iliac screws are also now commercially available (Fig. 11-7). Care should be taken to place the screw heads as far from the S1 screws, but as close in alignment with the rod trajectory as possible to minimize the need for offset connectors. Rod passage should proceed from cranial to caudal. This al-

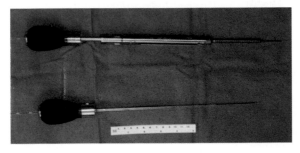

FIG. 11-7   Cannulated Viper 3-D 80 mm by 7.0 mm iliac screws and associated instruments.

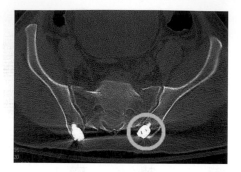

FIG. 11-8   CT scan demonstrating the importance of minimizing screw head prominence by recessing the polyaxial saddle below the PSIS.

lows better control of the iliac end of the rod tip to ensure proper articulation with the screw head (Fig. 11-8). It also allows the minimum amount of rod to extend past the screw head—otherwise there may be significant hardware prominence, which can cause local pain and cutaneous breakdown.

TRANSSACRAL SCREW FIXATION

Placing a fibula allograft shaft across the L5-S1 disc space through a sacral laminectomy has been well described for high-grade spondylolistheses.[4] More recently, a technique for accessing this route through a transsacral approach has been described. The incision is made near the base and to the right of the coccyx (for a right-handed surgeon). Blunt dissection is used to access the presacral fat pad for entry into the sacrum along the ventral aspect of its dome (Fig. 11-9). Drilling through the sacrum then allows access to the L5-S1 disc space and placement of a fixating implant across the disc space. A technique for two disc levels has been described more recently, and a differential thread pitch in the L5 and S1 components of the implant are designed to distract the disc space to improve foraminal height and spondylolistheses.

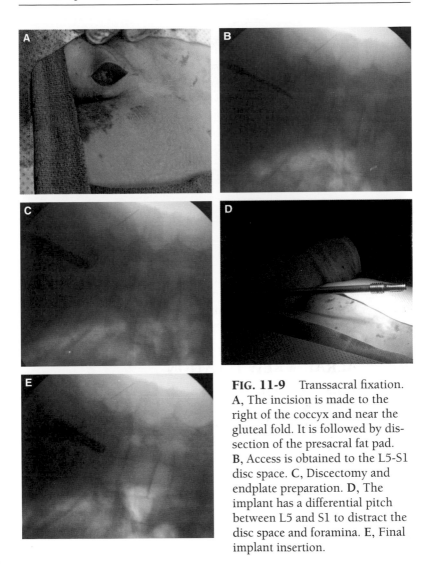

FIG. 11-9   Transsacral fixation. A, The incision is made to the right of the coccyx and near the gluteal fold. It is followed by dissection of the presacral fat pad. B, Access is obtained to the L5-S1 disc space. C, Discectomy and endplate preparation. D, The implant has a differential pitch between L5 and S1 to distract the disc space and foramina. E, Final implant insertion.

TRANSFACET SCREW FIXATION

The use of screws that span the facet joint is a truly percutaneous option for segmental fixation. Because the implant crosses the joint, fixation between the two vertebrae is accomplished with a single screw for each joint without connecting rods. Biomechanically, this method is inferior to pedicle screw–rod constructs, but if the spine is inherently stable and rigid, or if there are anterior

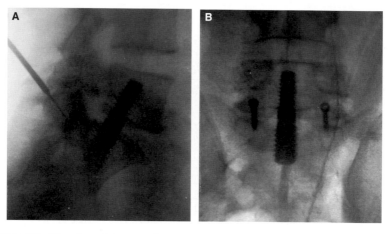

FIG. 11-10   A and B, Transfacet screws are placed through a cannulated percutaneous system at the L5-S1 level.

load-sharing constructs, it is a viable option (Fig. 11-10). Although translaminar facet screws have been in use for some time, the Bouchier technique, which directs the screw into the caudal pedicle, has become more popular, because it is easy to use and has a reduced risk of entry into the spinal canal.

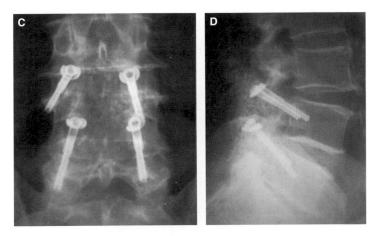

FIG. 11-10, cont'd   C and D, Screws are placed using the Bouchier technique; a screw/compression device is anchored in the pedicle of the caudal vertebral body.

MINIMALLY INVASIVE CROSS-LINKING

Transverse rod connectors allow for increased construct rigidity and are particularly useful for spinal deformity, osteoporosis, and asymmetric constructs. Cross connecting is also useful when fixation has been inadequate on only one side or when fixating areas of the spine prone to lateral bending or rotation. The major impediments to minimally invasive cross-linking are the spinous processes and interspinous ligaments. Any minimally invasive cross-link must span above the spinous processes, be passed between them, or include the removal of obstructing midline structures. Nevertheless, minimally invasive cross-linking can be achieved with a small footprint and low-profile instrumentation in select cases (Fig. 11-11).

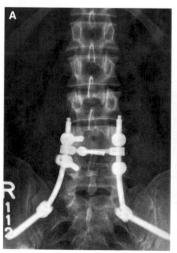
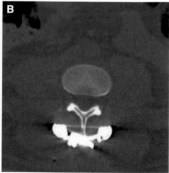

FIG. 11-11 A, Cross-links are placed to connect a percutaneous rod-screw system. In this example the interspinous ligament was partially removed. **B**, Notice that the implants are contoured and positioned dorsal to the lamina.

PERCUTANEOUS INTERBODY FUSION

Although still not completely validated, expandable interbody implants may offer an opportunity for disc space fusion through small access ports. Current minimally invasive TLIF options still require a significant incision and placement of grafts ranging from 8 to 14 mm in their largest linear dimension. The use of Kambin's triangle requires discectomy, endplate preparation, and placement of the cage through a 7 mm port or smaller. Such an approach has already been used successfully for endoscopic discectomy through small portals. Placing PEEK, titanium, and allograft-based interbody implants is already possible but still not widely accepted as achieving high fusion rates (Fig. 11-12). Successful arthrodesis will likely require the use of bone growth adjuvants, such as osteogenic substances or bone graft extenders.

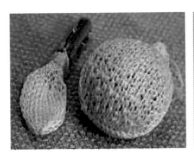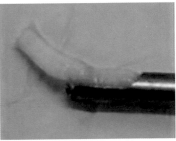

FIG. 11-12   OptiMesh expandable allograft-filled mesh bag (Spineology, Minneapolis, MN), which allows placement of a large-diameter interbody implant (18 to 25 mm) through a small port that is 7 mm in diameter.

MINIMALLY INVASIVE POSTEROLATERAL FUSION

Successful fusion using percutaneous surgery has typically involved arthrodesis in the interbody space. Although the posterolateral spine is a less robust fusion environment than the interbody space, for longer segment surgeries, or in the thoracic spine, posterolateral fusion may be more desirable. This is not only because of the inherent risks and complications associated with access of the interbody space at certain levels, but also because of the inefficiencies of performing more than three discectomies, endplate preparations, and graft placements.

Successful posterolateral intertransverse, lateral facet, or interlaminar fusion requires exposure of adequate bone surface area, which can be accomplished using a mini-open incision or speculum retractors (Fig. 11-13). We have found this technique to be most applicable in the lower thoracic region for a long-segment

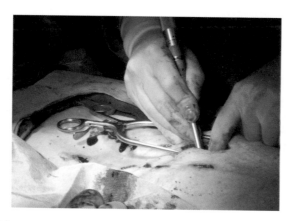

FIG. 11-13   Posterolateral fusion preparation of the lateral facet joints using a mini-open approach with drill decortications followed by placement of bone grafting adjuvants.

fusion spanning the thoracolumbar junction. Exposure of dorsal bone is followed by decortication with a high-speed burr and placement of bone graft, bone graft substitute, and/or bone graft extenders.

IMAGE-GUIDED TECHNOLOGY

Many surgeons prefer image guidance or frameless navigation to guide instrumentation placement for minimally invasive spine surgery. The obvious advantages include:
- Ease of use with real-time three-dimensional feedback on a computer screen
- Reduced intraoperative radiation exposure
- The ability to plan implant sizes and trajectories on the computer console
- Reduced operative times if the systems run efficiently

The drawbacks of these systems include:
- Capital equipment costs
- Technical problems
- Time for set-up and registration
- Reliance on technology that is prone to failure without bail-out options
- The potential to be misled with inaccurate or imprecise information in the absence of visible anatomic landmarks for confirmation.

Because of the drawbacks of image guidance, I prefer pedicle cannulation using fluoroscopy (see Chapter 3). Two-dimensional fluoroscopic imaging allows a surgeon to perform percutaneous fixation in even the most rudimentary of hospital settings and allows the surgeon to function even when technical issues arise with image guidance systems.

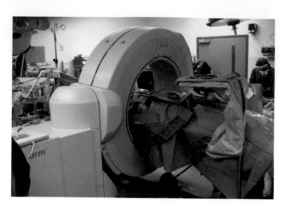

FIG. 11-14 Intraoperative three-dimensional imaging with an O-Arm (Medtronic Sofamor Danek USA, Memphis, TN), which is similar to CT scanning.

Because there are many systems currently available and their software and hardware packages are constantly evolving, I do not discuss any specific image guidance system here. However, the development of intraoperative three-dimensional imaging has allowed for confirmation of K-wire placement before final implant insertion.[5,6] This may prove particularly helpful in cases of deformity or revision, or when anatomic confines are limited such as with the upper lumbar pedicles (Fig. 11-14).

CONCLUSION

Minimally invasive spine surgery is still in its infancy. The range of minimally invasive techniques available will continue to expand and will likely soon include methods for osteotomy, severe deformity reduction, and posterolateral fusion of long constructs. Ultimately the goal is the duplication of the entire repertoire of traditional open surgery through less-invasive operations that cause the least disruption to the spine and its surrounding structures.

References

1. Amar A, Larsen D, Esnaashari N, et al. Percutaneous transpedicular polymethylmethacrylate vertebroplasty for the treatment of spinal compression fractures. Neurosurg 49:1105-1114, 2001.
2. Frankel B, D'Augustino S, Wang C. A biomechanical cadaveric analysis of polymethylmethacrylate-augmented pedicle screw fixation. J Neurosurg Spine 7:47-53, 2007.
3. Wang M, Ludwig S, Anderson G, et al. Percutaneous iliac screw placement: description of a new minimally invasive technique. Neurosurg Focus 25:1-5, 2008.
4. Smith J, Deviren V, Berven S, et al. Clinical outcome of trans-sacral interbody fusion after partial reduction for high-grade L5-S1 spondylolisthesis. Spine 26:2227-2234, 2001.
5. Nottmeier E, Young P. Image-guided placement of occipitocervical instrumentation using a reference arc attached to the headholder. Neurosurg 66(3 Suppl):S138-S142, 2010.
6. Wang M, Kim K, Liu C, et al. Reliability of 3-D fluoroscopy for detecting pedicle violations in the thoracic and lumbar spine. Neurosurg 54:1138-1143, 2004.

Index